The High-Fiber Kitchen Cookbook

Flavorful Recipes to Boost Digestive Health and Wellness

BY Terra Compasso

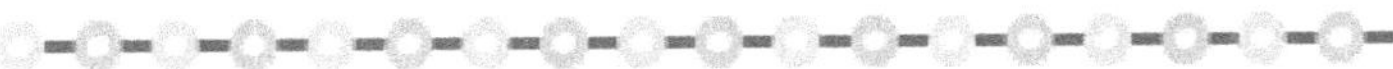

Licensing and Copyrighting

Table of Contents

Introduction

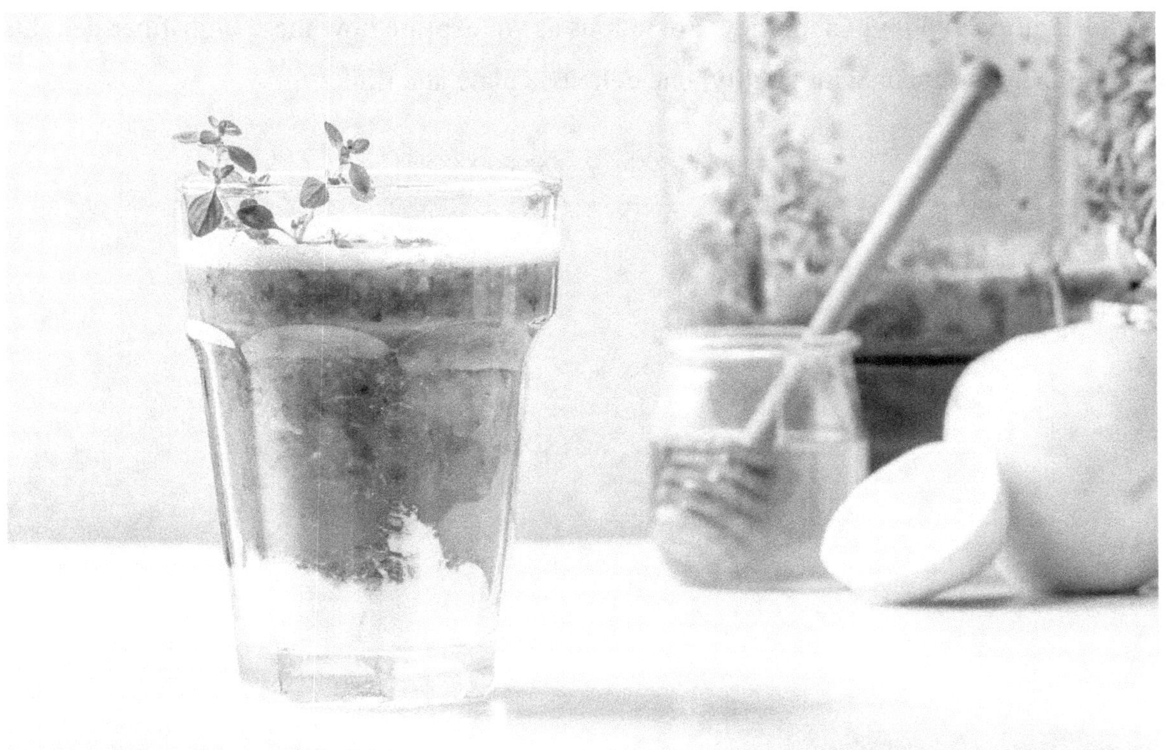

Welcome to the flavorful universe of Fiber-Rich Feasts, a culinary journey designed to not only tantalize your taste buds but also invigorate your well-being. Get ready to embark on a delectable adventure where health-conscious eating and scrumptious indulgence collide in harmony. Fiber-Rich Feasts aren't your typical health regimen; they're a celebration of vibrant colors, bold flavors, and the boundless possibilities that high-fiber ingredients offer. From the crunch of fresh vegetables to the hearty embrace of whole grains, every bite is a step toward nourishing your body while satisfying your cravings.

Beyond the confines of traditional notions about nutrition, Fiber-Rich Feasts open the door to a world of culinary creativity. Prepare to be delighted by inventive recipes that transform dietary essentials into culinary art, demonstrating that eating for wellness can be an exciting and joyous journey. So, join us as we explore how these high-fiber delights can infuse your meals with vitality, one delicious plate at a time.

XXXXXXXXXXXXXXXXXXX

1. Chia Pudding

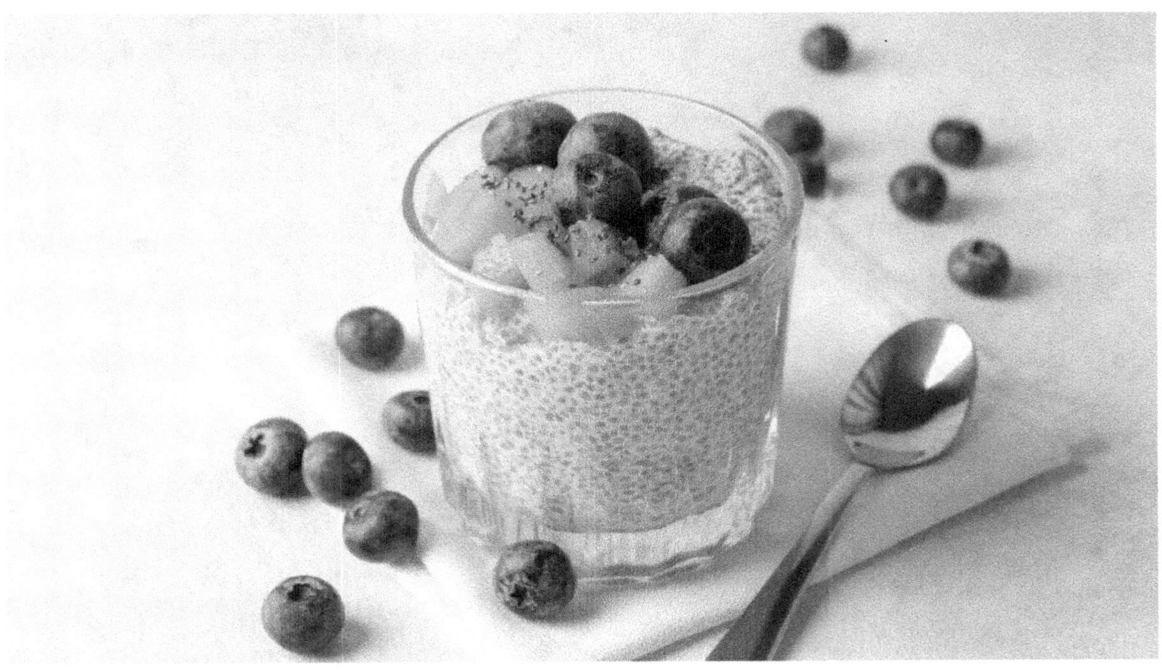

Chia Pudding is a nutritional delight. Tiny chia seeds absorb liquid to create a creamy, tapioca-like texture. With customizable flavors and toppings, it's a versatile and healthful option for breakfast or dessert, offering a satisfying blend of textures and a burst of energy in every spoonful.

Preparation Time: 15 minutes

Cook Time: 6 hours

Total Time: 6 hours 15 minutes

Serves: 4

Difficulty: Medium

Ingredients:

- 1/2 cup of chia seeds
- 2 cups of almond milk
- 4 tablespoons of maple syrup
- 1 teaspoon of vanilla extract
- 1/2 cup of fresh berries

Kitchen Tools Needed:

- Bowl
- Whisk
- Measuring Cups

xxxxxxxxxxxxxxxxxxx

Instructions:

a. Start by whisking together chia seeds, almond milk, maple syrup, and vanilla extract in a bowl. This will create the base of your chia pudding.

b. Allow the mixture to sit for 5 minutes. Afterward, give it another good whisk to ensure that there are no clumps and that all the ingredients are well combined.

c. Now, cover the bowl and place it in the refrigerator. Let it chill for at least 6 hours, or even better, leave it overnight. This resting period is essential as it allows the chia seeds to absorb the liquid and thicken, resulting in a creamy pudding-like texture.

d. Before serving, give the chia pudding a final stir to break up any clumps that may have formed during the chilling process.

e. To serve, divide the prepared chia pudding into 4 serving bowls or glasses.

f. Enhance the flavor and visual appeal by topping your chia pudding with an assortment of fresh berries. The burst of colors and fruity freshness adds a delightful contrast to the creamy pudding.

g. Your chia pudding is ready to be enjoyed. Serve it chilled, and savor the wholesome goodness.

Cooking Notes:

- Chia pudding is highly customizable. Feel free to experiment with various toppings like sliced bananas, chopped nuts, honey, or a sprinkle of cinnamon for added flavor and texture.
- Adjust the sweetness to your liking by varying the amount of maple syrup. Start with the recommended amount and add more if needed.
- Chia pudding can be made in larger batches and stored in the refrigerator for several days, making it a convenient option for meal prep or a quick breakfast.
- To make the pudding even creamier, you can use coconut milk or yogurt instead of almond milk.
- Don't rush the chilling process; allowing the pudding to rest for an adequate amount of time is essential for achieving the desired consistency.

2. Perfect Bowl of Oats

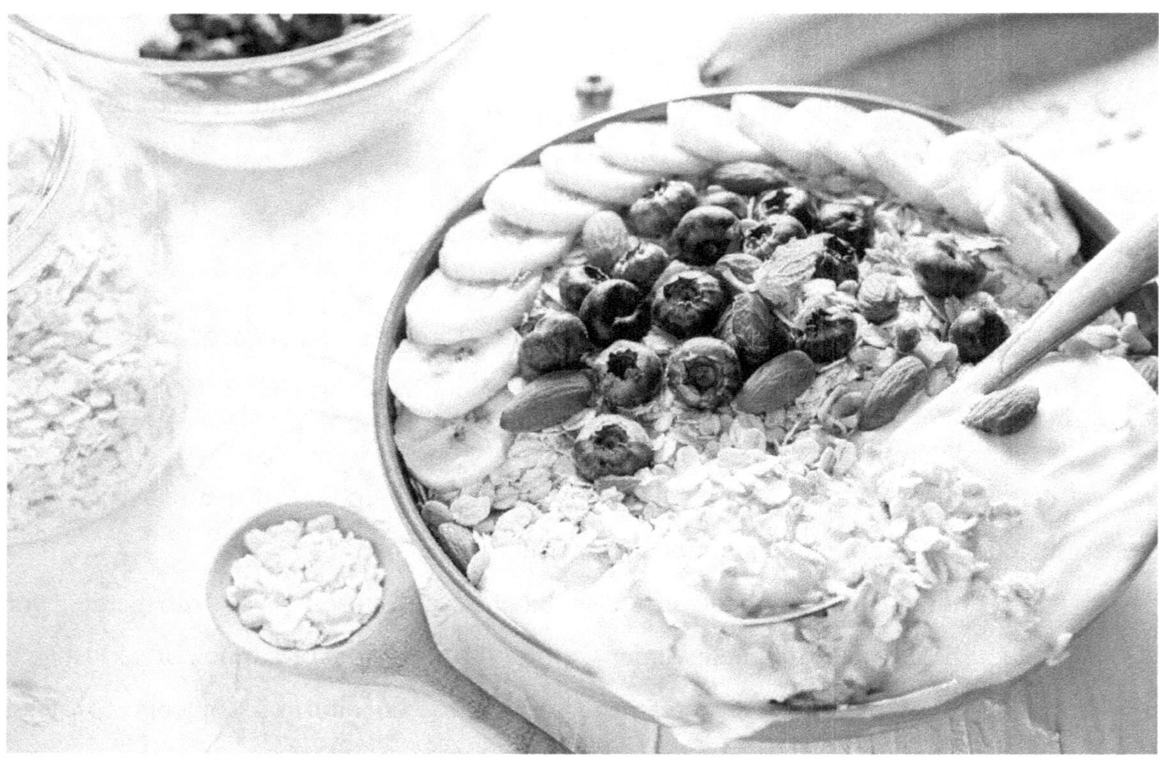

The Perfect Bowl of Oats is a comforting classic. Creamy, cooked oats meet a variety of toppings—fruits, nuts, and honey—for a balanced and nourishing start to the day. It's a warm and hearty option that offers both indulgence and sustenance in a single bowl.

Preparation Time: 15 minutes

Cook Time: 6 hours

Total Time: 6 hours 15 minutes

Serves: 2

Difficulty: Medium

Ingredients:

- 1 cup of rolled oats
- 2 cups of water
- 1 cup of almond milk
- 2 tablespoons of maple syrup
- 1/4 teaspoon of cinnamon
- 1/4 cup of sliced strawberries
- 1/4 cup of blueberries
- 2 tablespoons of chopped almonds

Kitchen Tools Needed:

- saucepan
- spoon
- bowl

XXXXXXXXXXXXXXXXXXXX

Instructions:

a. Start by preparing a delicious bowl of oats. In a saucepan, combine the rolled oats, water, almond milk, maple syrup, and a pinch of cinnamon. These ingredients will come together to create a hearty and flavorful oatmeal base.

b. Over medium heat, bring this mixture to a gentle boil. Once it's reached a boil, reduce the heat to low and continue cooking. Stir regularly to ensure the oats cook evenly and absorb all the delicious flavors. This simmering process should take around 15 minutes.

c. Keep an eye on the oats. You'll know they're ready when they turn creamy and tender, creating a comforting and satisfying texture.

d. Remove the saucepan from the heat once the oats have achieved the desired consistency.

e. Now, it's time to serve up your perfect bowl of oats. Divide the oatmeal evenly into two bowls, ensuring that each serving is equally delicious.

f. For the finishing touches, adorn each bowl with slices of fresh, vibrant strawberries, juicy blueberries, and a generous sprinkle of chopped almonds. These toppings not only add delightful flavors but also provide a satisfying contrast of textures.

g. Your perfect bowl of oats is ready to be enjoyed. Serve it warm, savor every spoonful, and relish in the comforting goodness of this delightful breakfast treat.

Cooking Notes:

- Customize your oatmeal by experimenting with different toppings such as sliced bananas, diced apples, a drizzle of honey, or a dollop of yogurt for added creaminess.

- Adjust the sweetness to your liking. If you prefer a sweeter oatmeal, simply add more maple syrup or a sweetener of your choice.

- To make this recipe even more nutritious, consider incorporating superfoods like chia seeds, flaxseeds, or a scoop of protein powder for an extra energy boost.

- If you're short on time in the morning, you can prepare the oatmeal base the night before and simply reheat it when you're ready to enjoy it. This way, you can have a satisfying and nutritious breakfast in minutes.

- Don't hesitate to experiment with different spices like nutmeg, vanilla extract, or a pinch of cardamom to add unique flavors to your oatmeal.

3. Peanut Butter Overnight Oats

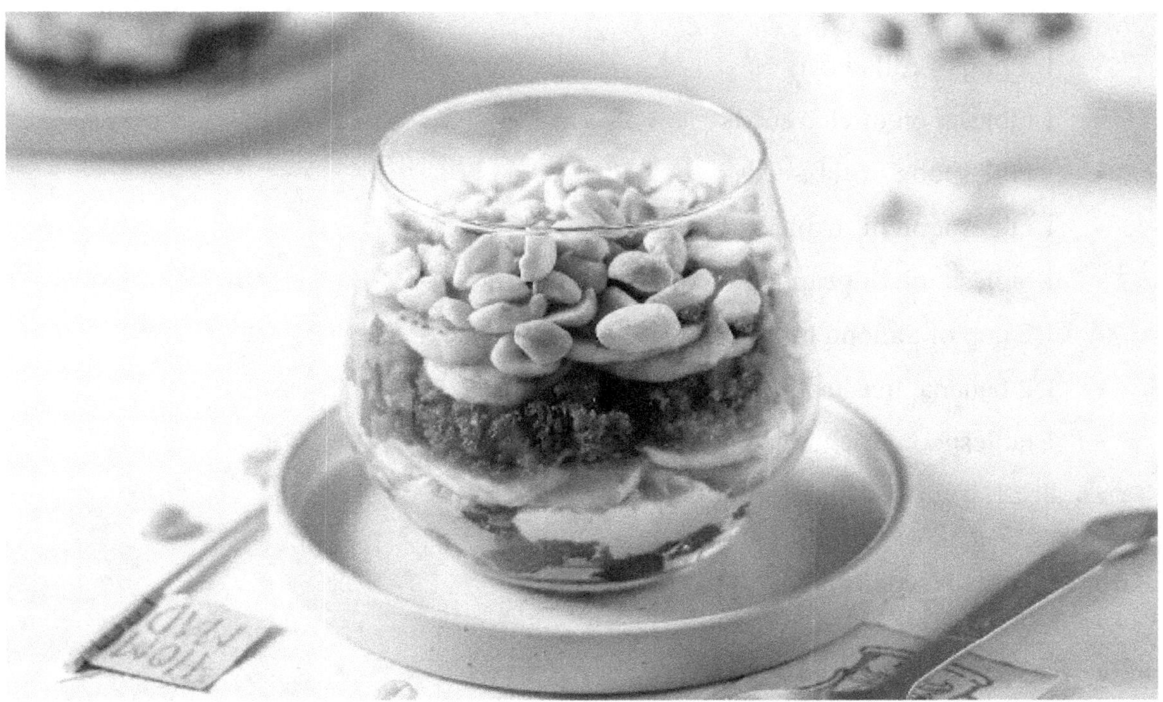

Peanut Butter Overnight Oats offer morning ease. Rolled oats soak in nutty goodness, mixed with creamy peanut butter and milk. Refrigerated overnight, it's a ready-to-enjoy breakfast with a satisfying blend of textures and flavors, providing a convenient and energizing start to the day.

Preparation Time: 15 minutes

Cook Time: 6 hours

Total Time: 6 hours 15 minutes

Serves: 1

Difficulty: Medium

Ingredients:

- 1/2 cup of rolled oats
- 1 tablespoon of chia seeds
- 1 tablespoon of flaxseeds
- 1 tablespoon of maple syrup
- 1 tablespoon of peanut butter
- 1/2 cup of almond milk
- 1/2 banana, mashed
- 1 tablespoon of chopped peanuts
- Fresh fruit for topping (optional)

Kitchen Tools Needed:

- saucepan
- spoon
- bowl

XXXXXXXXXXXXXXXXXXXX

Instructions:

a. Begin by gathering all your ingredients for this delightful breakfast.

b. In a mason jar or any container with a lid, combine the rolled oats, chia seeds, flaxseeds, maple syrup, peanut butter, almond milk, and mashed banana. These ingredients together create a nourishing and delicious base for your overnight oats.

c. Stir everything thoroughly, making sure that all components are well mixed. This ensures that the oats and seeds absorb the liquid evenly, giving you a creamy and satisfying texture.

d. Once everything is mixed to your satisfaction, securely cover the mason jar or container. This step is crucial as it allows the oats and seeds to soak and soften overnight, infusing them with all those delightful flavors.

e. Now, it's time to be patient and let your mixture work its magic. Refrigerate it overnight or for a minimum of 6 hours. This resting period allows the oats and seeds to absorb the liquid, creating that creamy and luscious consistency that makes overnight oats so irresistible.

f. When you're ready to enjoy your Peanut Butter Overnight Oats, give the mixture a good stir. This step ensures that the peanut butter, banana, and all the other delightful ingredients are evenly distributed.

g. To add a delightful crunch and burst of flavor, top your oats with chopped peanuts and fresh fruit, if desired. This step not only adds texture and visual appeal but also complements the creamy oats perfectly.

h. Now, dig in and savor your Peanut Butter Overnight Oats. The combination of peanut butter, banana, and maple syrup creates a sweet and nutty flavor profile that's simply delicious.

Cooking Notes:

- Feel free to adjust the sweetness to your liking by adding more or less maple syrup.
- Experiment with different toppings. Fresh berries, sliced banana, a drizzle of honey, or a sprinkle of cocoa nibs can all make your overnight oats extra special.
- If you're in a rush, you can prepare this breakfast in the morning and let it chill in the fridge while you get ready.
- Overnight oats are incredibly versatile. Try adding a scoop of protein powder or a dollop of yogurt for extra creaminess and protein.
- Make a batch of these oats at the beginning of the week for a quick and easy breakfast option on busy mornings.

4. Cozy Turmeric Porridge

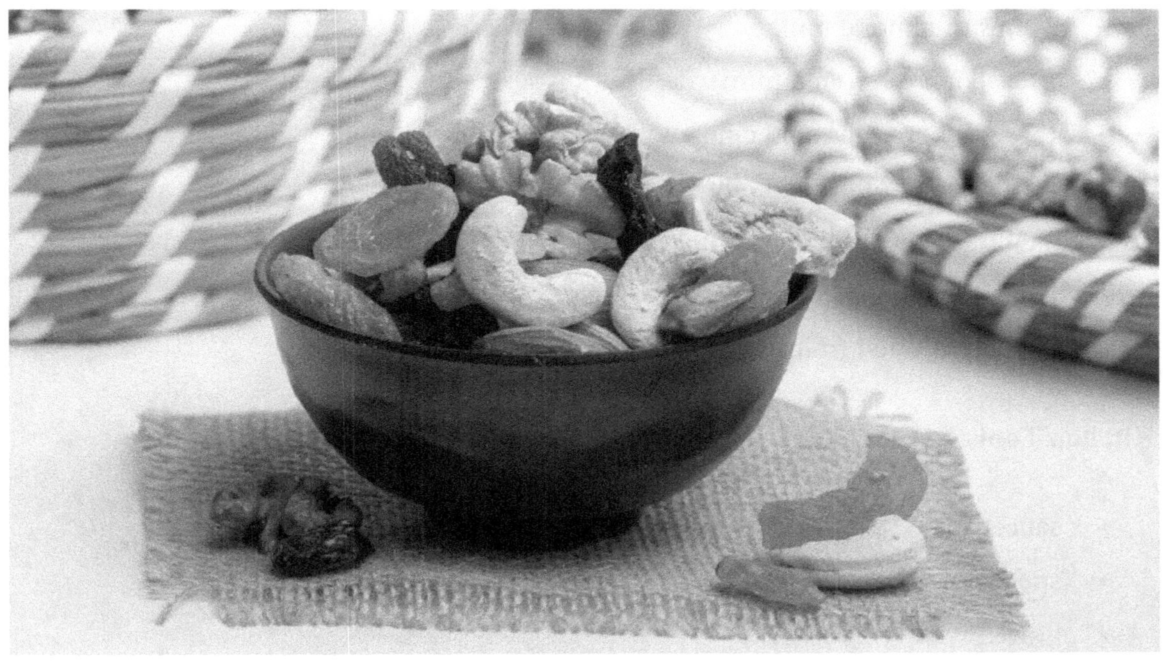

Cozy Turmeric Porridge is a warm embrace. Creamy oats infused with turmeric's warmth create a comforting base. Topped with nuts, spices, and a drizzle of honey, it's a flavorful and aromatic bowl that offers both nourishment and a soothing start to the day.

Preparation Time: 15 minutes

Cook Time: 6 hours

Total Time: 6 hours 15 minutes

Serves: 2

Difficulty: Medium

Ingredients:

- 1 cup of rolled oats
- 2 cups of almond milk
- 1 teaspoon of ground turmeric
- 1/2 teaspoon of ground cinnamon
- 1/4 teaspoon of ground ginger
- 2 tablespoons of maple syrup
- 1/4 cup of chopped nuts
- 1/4 cup of dried fruits

Kitchen Tools Needed:

- saucepan
- spoon
- bowl

XXXXXXXXXXXXXXXXXXXX

Instructions:

a. Start by combining rolled oats, almond milk, ground turmeric, cinnamon, and ginger in a saucepan. These ingredients will infuse your porridge with warm and cozy flavors.

b. Over medium heat, bring the mixture to a gentle boil. Stirring occasionally ensures that the spices are evenly distributed, creating a delicious and aromatic base.

c. Once it reaches a boil, reduce the heat to low. Continue to simmer and stir occasionally for approximately 10-15 minutes. This allows the oats to cook until tender, and the porridge achieves the desired thickness.

d. Add maple syrup to the porridge and mix it in. This natural sweetener enhances the flavor and sweetness of your cozy turmeric porridge.

e. Remove the saucepan from heat and let the porridge cool for a few minutes. This cooling step ensures a safe temperature for consumption.

f. Divide the warm and fragrant porridge into two bowls. This recipe yields two servings, making it perfect for sharing or saving one for later.

g. Elevate your cozy turmeric porridge by topping it with a generous handful of chopped nuts and dried fruits. These toppings add both texture and a burst of additional flavors.

h. Serve your heartwarming creation while it's still warm, savoring the delightful blend of spices and the comforting appeal of this turmeric-infused porridge.

Cooking Notes:

- Adjust the sweetness to your liking by adding more or less maple syrup. You can also substitute it with honey or any sweetener of your choice.
- Feel free to experiment with the toppings. Sliced bananas, fresh berries, or a dollop of yogurt can complement the flavors and textures of your porridge.
- Turmeric can stain, so be cautious when handling it, especially on clothing and countertops.
- Turmeric has a bold flavor, so you can adjust the amount to suit your taste preferences.
- This porridge is not only delicious but also packed with anti-inflammatory properties from the turmeric and ginger, making it a nutritious and comforting breakfast option.

5. Vegan Whole Grain Waffles with Roasted Stone Fruit

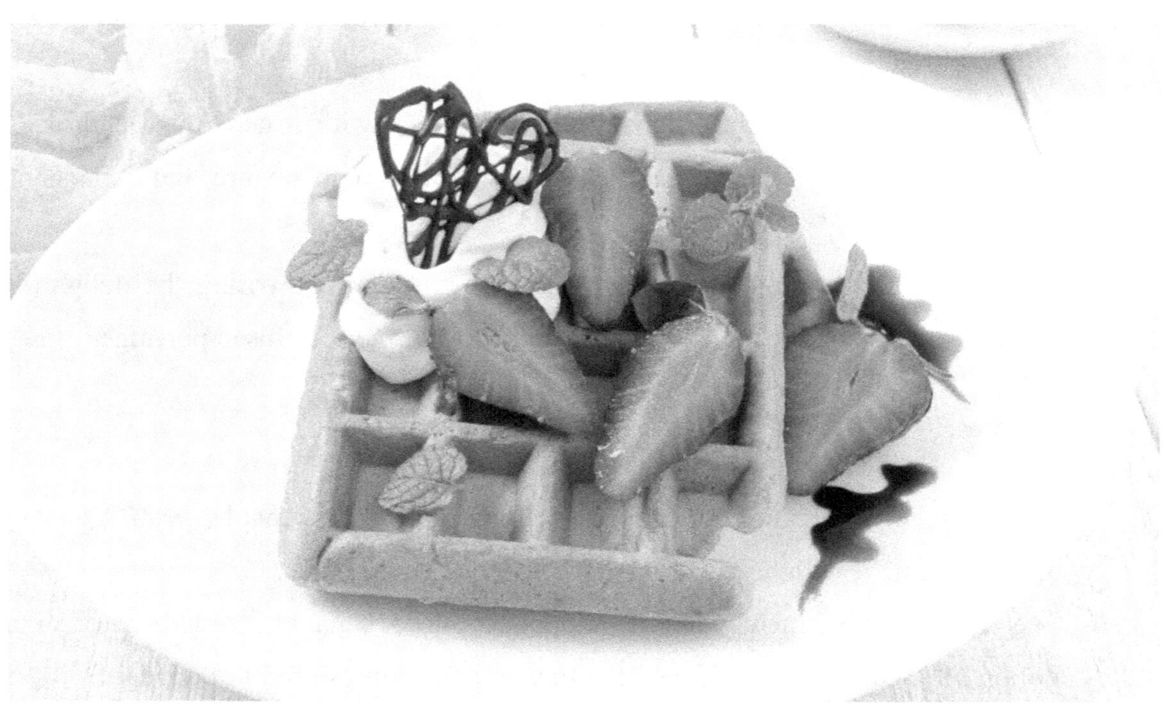

Vegan Whole Grain Waffles with Roasted Stone Fruit redefine breakfast. Nutty whole-grain waffles are topped with lusciously roasted stone fruits, offering a delightful blend of flavors and textures. This plant-based indulgence creates a colorful and satisfying start to the day that celebrates both taste and wholesomeness.

Preparation Time: 10 minutes

Cook Time: 35 minutes

Total Time: 45 minutes

Serves: 3

Difficulty: Medium

Ingredients:

- 2 cups of whole wheat flour
- 1/2 cup of rolled oats
- 2 tablespoons of ground flaxseed
- 2 teaspoons of baking powder
- 1/2 teaspoon of baking soda
- 1/4 teaspoon of salt
- 2 cups of almond milk
- 2 tablespoons of maple syrup
- 1 teaspoon of vanilla extract
- 2 peaches, sliced
- 2 plums, sliced
- 1 tablespoon of coconut oil
- 1 tablespoon of maple syrup
- 1/4 teaspoon of cinnamon

Kitchen Tools Needed:

- waffle iron
- oven
- mixing bowl
- whisk
- baking sheet

xxxxxxxxxxxxxxxxxxx

Instructions:

a. Begin by preheating your waffle iron, ensuring it's hot and ready for cooking.

b. In a mixing bowl, combine whole wheat flour, rolled oats, ground flaxseed, baking powder, baking soda, and a pinch of salt. Whisk these dry ingredients together to form the waffle batter base.

c. To the dry mixture, add almond milk, maple syrup, and a dash of vanilla extract. Stir thoroughly until all the ingredients are well incorporated, forming a smooth batter.

d. Carefully pour the batter onto your preheated waffle iron. Use the recommended amount of batter for your specific waffle iron to ensure consistent results.

e. Close the waffle iron and let the waffles cook until they turn a lovely shade of golden brown and develop a crispy texture.

f. Now, let's prepare the delicious roasted stone fruit. Preheat your oven to 400°F (200°C) in preparation for this step.

g. On a baking sheet, artfully arrange slices of peaches and plums. Drizzle them with a touch of coconut oil and a drizzle of maple syrup. To enhance the flavors, sprinkle a pinch of cinnamon over the fruit.

h. Roast this delightful fruit medley in the oven for approximately 15 minutes. Keep a close eye on them, as you want the fruits to turn soft and acquire a beautiful caramelized finish.

i. Once your waffles and roasted stone fruit are ready, it's time to serve. Place the vegan whole grain waffles on a plate and generously top them with the caramelized roasted stone fruit.

j. Savor the delightful combination of flavors and textures as you enjoy your vegan whole grain waffles with roasted stone fruit.

Cooking Notes:

- Adjust the sweetness to your liking by varying the amount of maple syrup in the waffle batter.
- Experiment with different stone fruits depending on what's in season or your personal preferences.
- Top your waffles with a dollop of dairy-free yogurt or a sprinkle of chopped nuts for added variety.
- Leftover waffles and roasted fruit can be refrigerated and reheated for a quick and satisfying breakfast another day.
- Feel free to explore various spices like nutmeg or cardamom to further enhance the roasted fruit's flavor.

6. Super Seedy Granola Bars

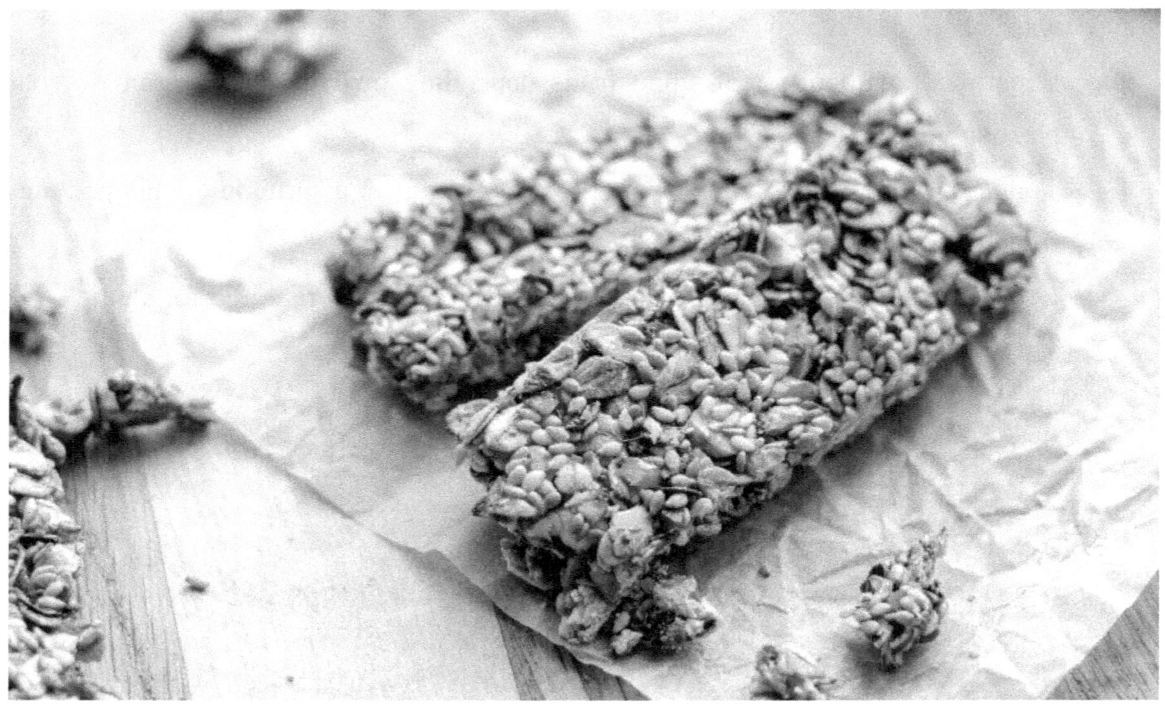

Super Seedy Granola Bars offer a nutritious energy boost. Packed with a medley of seeds, oats, and dried fruits, they provide a satisfying crunch. These homemade bars are a wholesome and convenient snack that delivers a blend of textures and flavors, perfect for a quick and nourishing pick-me-up.

Preparation Time: 10 minutes

Cook Time: 35 minutes

Total Time: 45 minutes

Serves: 10

Difficulty: Medium

Ingredients:

- 1 cup of rolled oats
- 1/2 cup of unsweetened shredded coconut
- 1/2 cup of pumpkin seeds
- 1/2 cup of sunflower seeds
- 1/2 cup of flaxseeds
- 1/2 cup of chia seeds
- 1/2 cup of chopped almonds
- 1/2 cup of chopped dried cranberries
- 1/2 cup of honey
- 1/4 cup of almond butter
- 1/4 cup of coconut oil
- 1 teaspoon of vanilla extract
- 1/2 teaspoon of cinnamon
- 1/4 teaspoon of salt

Kitchen Tools Needed:

- Mixing bowl
- Baking dish
- Parchment paper
- Spatula

xxxxxxxxxxxxxxxxxxxx

Instructions:

a. Preheat your oven to 350°F (175°C).

b. In a mixing bowl, combine rolled oats, shredded coconut, pumpkin seeds, sunflower seeds, flaxseeds, chia seeds, chopped almonds, and dried cranberries.

c. In a small saucepan, heat honey, almond butter, coconut oil, vanilla extract, cinnamon, and salt over low heat until they're melted and well mixed.

d. Pour the melted mixture over the dry ingredients and mix thoroughly until everything is evenly coated.

e. Line a baking dish with parchment paper and press the mixture firmly into the dish.

f. Bake in the preheated oven for 20-25 minutes, or until it turns golden brown. Remove it from the oven and let it cool completely before slicing it into bars.

g. You can store these bars in an airtight container in the refrigerator for up to 2 weeks.

Cooking Notes:

- Customize your granola bars by adding your favorite nuts, seeds, or dried fruits.
- Be sure to press the mixture firmly into the baking dish to help the bars hold together.
- If you prefer sweeter bars, you can increase the amount of honey or add a sweetener of your choice.
- To make the bars gluten-free, use certified gluten-free oats and double-check that all your ingredients are gluten-free.
- Feel free to experiment with different flavors by adding spices like nutmeg or cardamom to the mixture.

7. Healthy Brownie Granola Bars

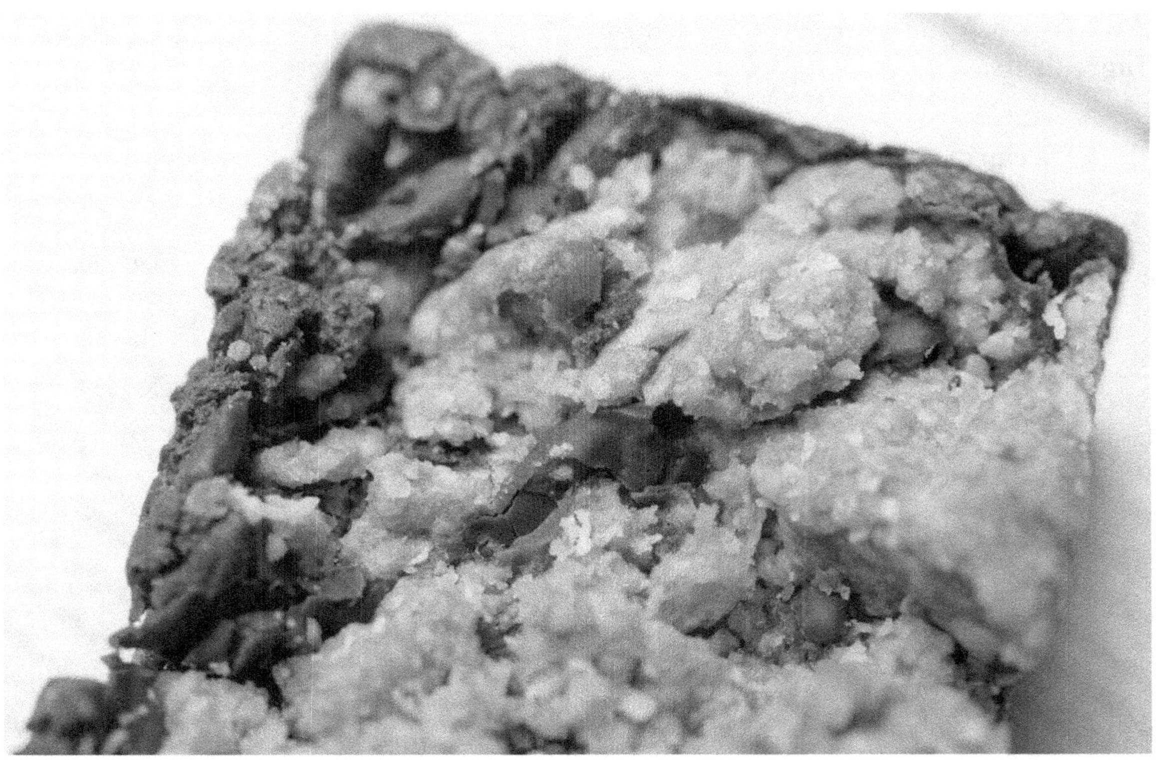

Healthy Brownie Granola Bars redefine indulgence. Rich, chocolaty flavors meet a medley of wholesome ingredients like nuts, oats, and dates. These guilt-free bars offer a chewy and satisfying treat, combining the allure of brownies with the goodness of nutritious ingredients in every bite.

Preparation Time: 10 minutes

Cook Time: 35 minutes

Total Time: 45 minutes

Serves: 12

Difficulty: Medium

Ingredients:

- 1 cup of oats
- 1/2 cup of almond butter
- 14 cups of honey
- 1/4 cup of unsweetened cocoa powder
- 1/4 cup of dark chocolate chips
- 1/4 cup of dried cranberries
- 1/4 cup of chopped almonds
- 1/4 cup of flaxseeds
- 1 teaspoon of vanilla extract
- A pinch of salt

Kitchen Tools Needed:

- Baking dish
- Mixing bowl
- Whisk

xxxxxxxxxxxxxxxxxxxx

Instructions:

a. Preheat your oven to 350°F (175°C) and line a baking dish with parchment paper for easy removal later.

b. In a mixing bowl, combine the almond butter, honey, cocoa powder, vanilla extract, and a pinch of salt. Make sure to mix these ingredients thoroughly.

c. Add the oats, dark chocolate chips, dried cranberries, chopped almonds, and flaxseeds to the mixture. Stir until all the ingredients are well combined, creating a delicious and nutritious base.

d. Transfer this mixture into the prepared baking dish, and use a spatula or your hands to press it down evenly, ensuring it's compact.

e. Bake in the preheated oven for approximately 15-20 minutes. Keep an eye on it and remove it when the edges turn slightly browned.

f. Take it out of the oven and allow it to cool completely right in the baking dish.

g. Once it's cool, cut it into 12 bars, and they're ready to enjoy!

Cooking Notes:

- You can get creative with your add-ins. Consider using other nuts, seeds, or dried fruits like raisins or apricots for variety.

- To make these bars vegan, replace honey with maple syrup or agave nectar.

- Store your brownie granola bars in an airtight container at room temperature for up to a week. If you want them to last longer, keep them in the fridge.

- These bars are great for on-the-go snacks, but if you're planning to pack them, you can individually wrap them in parchment paper for convenience.

- Feel free to adjust the sweetness by adding more honey or cocoa powder to suit your taste.

8. Creamy Pineapple Cucumber Smoothie

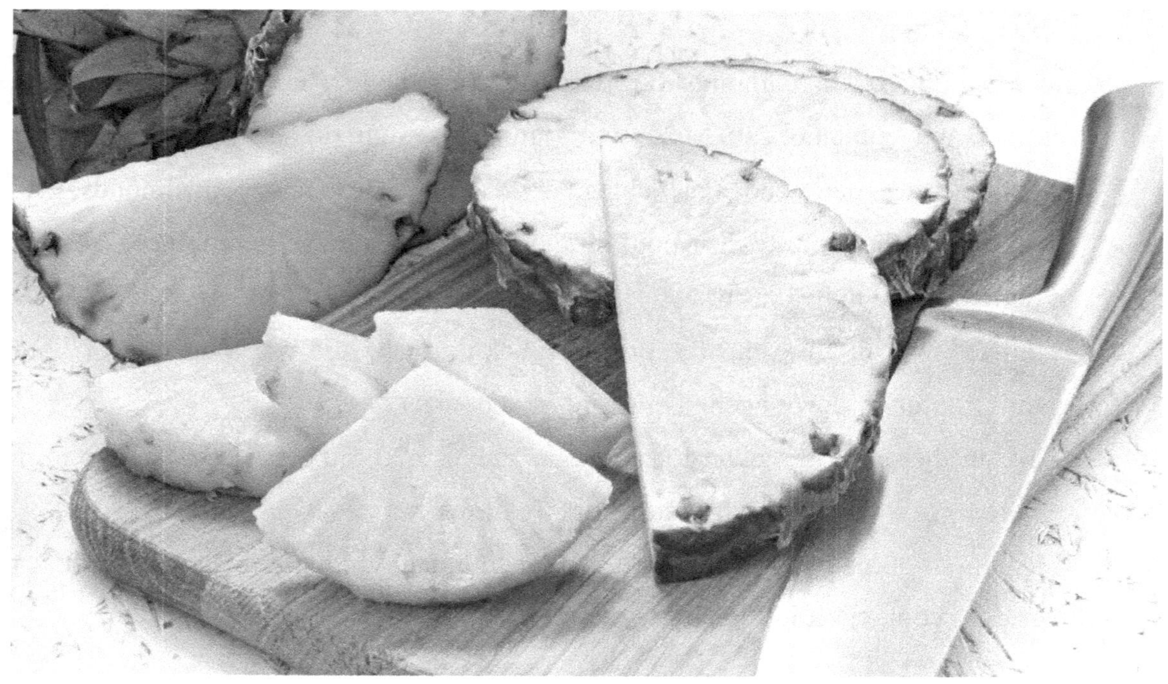

Creamy Pineapple Cucumber Smoothie refreshes the senses. Blending the sweetness of pineapple with the coolness of cucumber, it's a tropical delight. With a creamy base, this revitalizing smoothie offers a balance of flavors that's both invigorating and hydrating—a perfect sip to brighten your day.

Preparation Time: 10 minutes

Cook Time: 35 minutes

Total Time: 45 minutes

Serves: 1

Difficulty: Medium

Ingredients:

- 1 cup of pineapple chunks
- 1/2 cup of cucumber
- 1/2 cup of Greek yogurt
- 1/2 cup of coconut milk
- 1 tablespoon of honey
- Ice cubes

Kitchen Tools Needed:

- Blender

xxxxxxxxxxxxxxxxxxxx

Instructions:

a. Begin by peeling and chopping the cucumber into small, manageable pieces.
b. In a blender, combine the pineapple chunks, chopped cucumber, Greek yogurt, coconut milk, honey, and ice cubes.
c. Blend these ingredients together until you achieve a smooth and creamy texture.
d. Once your creamy pineapple cucumber smoothie is perfectly blended, pour it into a chilled glass.
e. Serve and enjoy your refreshing creation!

Cooking Notes:

- Adjust the sweetness to your liking by adding more or less honey.
- If you prefer a thicker consistency, consider using frozen pineapple chunks or adding more ice cubes.
- For an extra nutritional boost, toss in a handful of spinach or kale. It won't alter the flavor significantly and adds valuable vitamins.
- Don't hesitate to experiment with different fruits or add a touch of fresh mint for a delightful twist.
- This smoothie is best enjoyed immediately to savor its freshness, but you can store any leftovers in the refrigerator for a short time.

9. Gingery Mango & Berry Smoothie

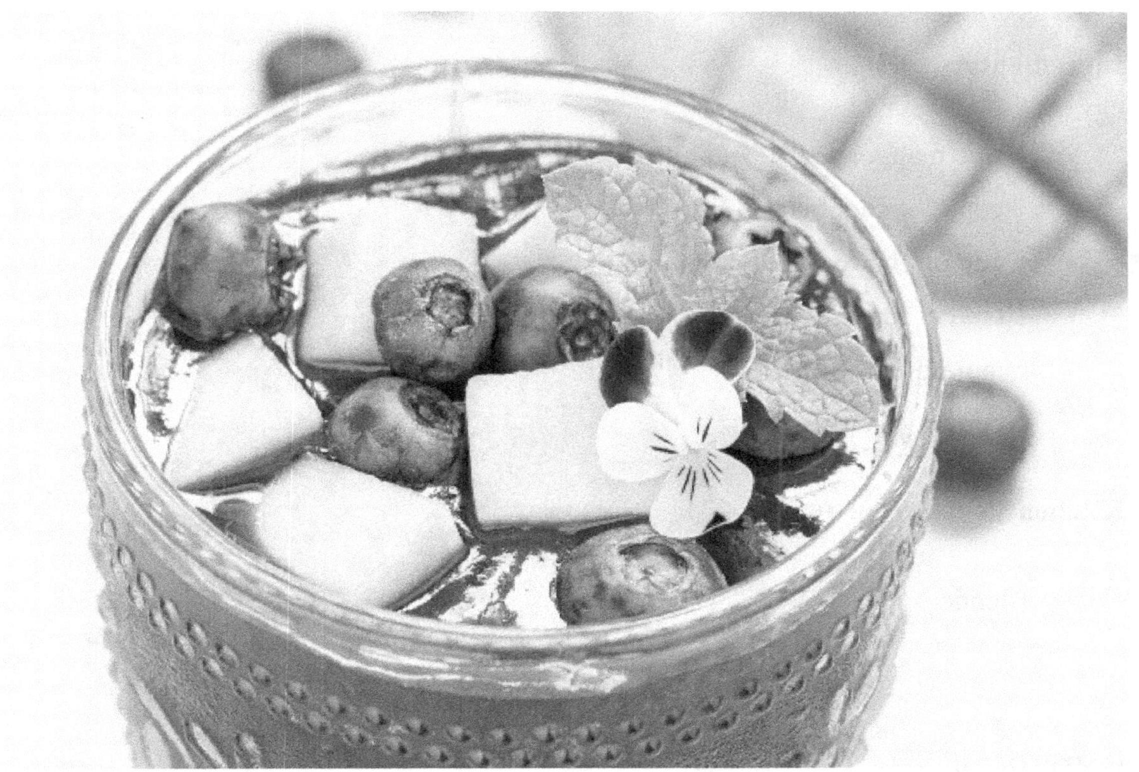

Gingery Mango & Berry Smoothie brings a zing of flavor. Juicy mango and vibrant berries meet the warmth of ginger, creating a refreshing and aromatic blend. With a touch of tang and spice, this smoothie offers a delightful fusion that's both invigorating and satisfying for a fruity treat.

Preparation Time: 10 minutes

Cook Time: 35 minutes

Total Time: 45 minutes

Serves: 2

Difficulty: Medium

Ingredients:

- 1 ripe mango, peeled and pitted
- 1 cup of mixed berries
- 1 cup of unsweetened almond milk
- 1 tablespoon of grated fresh ginger
- 2 tablespoons of honey
- 1 cup of ice cubes

Kitchen Tools Needed:

- Blender

XXXXXXXXXXXXXXXXXXX

Instructions:

a. In a blender, add ripe mango, a mix of berries (such as strawberries, blueberries, and raspberries), almond milk, fresh ginger, honey, and ice cubes.
b. Blend until all the ingredients are thoroughly combined, creating a smooth and creamy texture.
c. Carefully pour the vibrant smoothie into glasses.
d. Serve the refreshing Gingery Mango & Berry Smoothie chilled and enjoy!

Cooking Notes:

- Adjust the sweetness by adding more or less honey, depending on your taste preferences.
- For an extra frosty texture, consider using frozen mixed berries instead of fresh ones, reducing the need for additional ice cubes.
- Feel free to swap almond milk with your preferred milk or dairy-free alternative.
- Experiment with different fruits or additional spices like cinnamon for unique flavor profiles.
- To make it a more substantial meal, consider adding a scoop of protein powder, a dollop of Greek yogurt, or some oats for added nutrition and satiety.
- Prepare extra servings and freeze them in popsicle molds for a delightful summer treat.

10. Superfoods Green Lemonade Smoothie

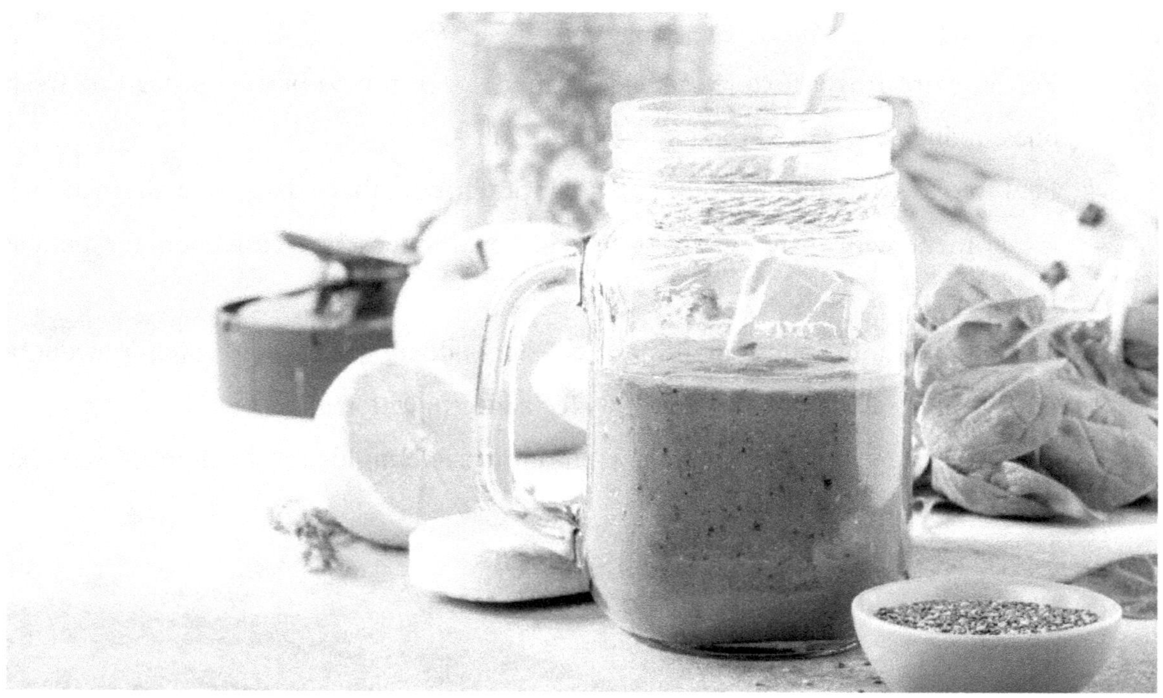

Superfoods Green Lemonade Smoothie is a zesty boost. Packed with nutrient-rich greens, like spinach and kale, it's blended with lemon for a tangy kick. With chia seeds and other superfoods, this vibrant smoothie offers a revitalizing and healthful sip that's both refreshing and nourishing.

Preparation Time: 10 minutes

Cook Time: 35 minutes

Total Time: 45 minutes

Serves: 2

Difficulty: Medium

Ingredients:

- 2 cups of spinach leaves
- 1 cup of kale leaves
- 1 ripe avocado
- 1 green apple
- 1 cucumber
- 1 lemon, juiced
- 1 tablespoon of chia seeds
- 1 tablespoon of honey
- 2 cups of almond milk

Kitchen Tools Needed:

- Blender

XXXXXXXXXXXXXXXXXXX

Instructions:

a. Begin by thoroughly washing the spinach and kale leaves to remove any impurities.

b. Peel and pit the avocado, then cut it into manageable chunks.

c. Core the green apple and slice it into rings.

d. For the cucumber, peel it, remove the seeds, and cut it into chunks.

e. Now, in your trusty blender, add the washed spinach and kale leaves, the prepared avocado, sliced green apple, cucumber chunks, freshly squeezed lemon juice, chia seeds, honey, and almond milk.

f. Blend all these vibrant ingredients until they merge into a smooth and creamy consistency.

g. Finally, pour your Superfoods Green Lemonade Smoothie into glasses and serve it refreshingly chilled.

Cooking Notes:

- If you prefer a thicker smoothie, consider adding ice cubes to the blender before blending.
- Customize your smoothie by adjusting the sweetness level with more or less honey as desired.
- For an extra nutritional boost, you can incorporate other superfood ingredients like spirulina, flaxseeds, or a scoop of plant-based protein powder.
- To make this smoothie even more filling, try adding a spoonful of Greek yogurt or a handful of rolled oats for added creaminess and texture.

11. PB&J Smoothie

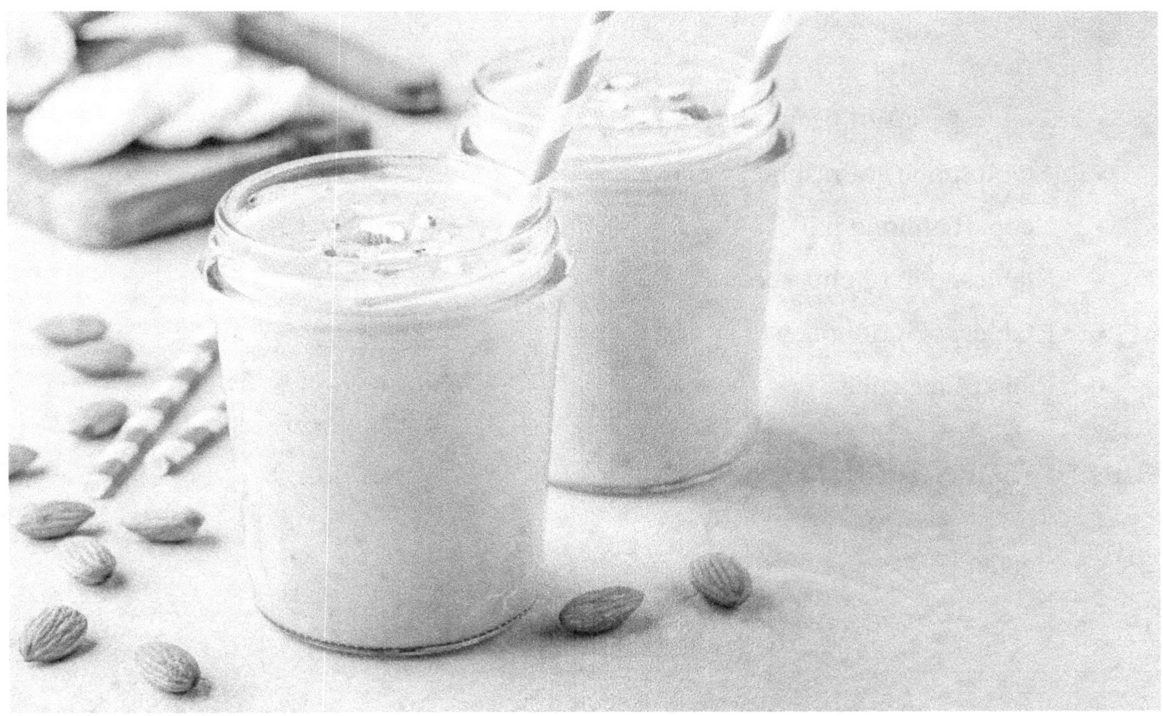

PB&J Smoothie revives a classic combo. Creamy peanut butter and sweet berry goodness blend harmoniously, capturing the essence of a favorite sandwich. With a protein punch and fruity delight, this smoothie is a nostalgic yet nutritious treat that's perfect for a satisfying sip any time of day.

Preparation Time: 10 minutes

Cook Time: 55 minutes

Total Time: 1 hour 5 minutes

Serves: 2

Difficulty: Medium

Ingredients:

- 2 ripe bananas
- 2 tablespoons of peanut butter
- 2 tablespoons of raspberry jam
- 1 cup of almond milk
- 1 tablespoon of chia seeds
- 1 tablespoon of honey
- 1 cup of ice cubes

Kitchen Tools Needed:

- blender

xxxxxxxxxxxxxxxxxxxx

Instructions:

a. Start by peeling and slicing the bananas into manageable pieces.
b. In a blender, combine the sliced bananas, peanut butter, raspberry jam, almond milk, chia seeds, honey, and ice cubes.
c. Blend all these ingredients on high speed until the mixture achieves a smooth and creamy consistency.
d. Carefully pour the luscious smoothie into glasses, ensuring an even distribution, and serve it refreshingly chilled.

Cooking Notes:

- Customize your PB&J Smoothie by experimenting with different types of nut butter, such as almond or cashew butter, for unique flavors and textures.
- Adjust the sweetness to your liking by varying the amount of honey or choosing between regular, reduced-sugar, or no-sugar-added raspberry jam.
- If you prefer a thicker smoothie, you can add more ice cubes or a frozen banana for a frostier consistency.
- For added nutrition and a fiber boost, consider adding a handful of spinach or kale leaves to the blend; you'll hardly notice the greens amidst the delicious flavors.
- Leftover smoothie can be stored in an airtight container in the refrigerator for a short time. However, it's best enjoyed fresh to maintain its optimal taste and texture.

12. Chipotle Tofu Chilaquiles

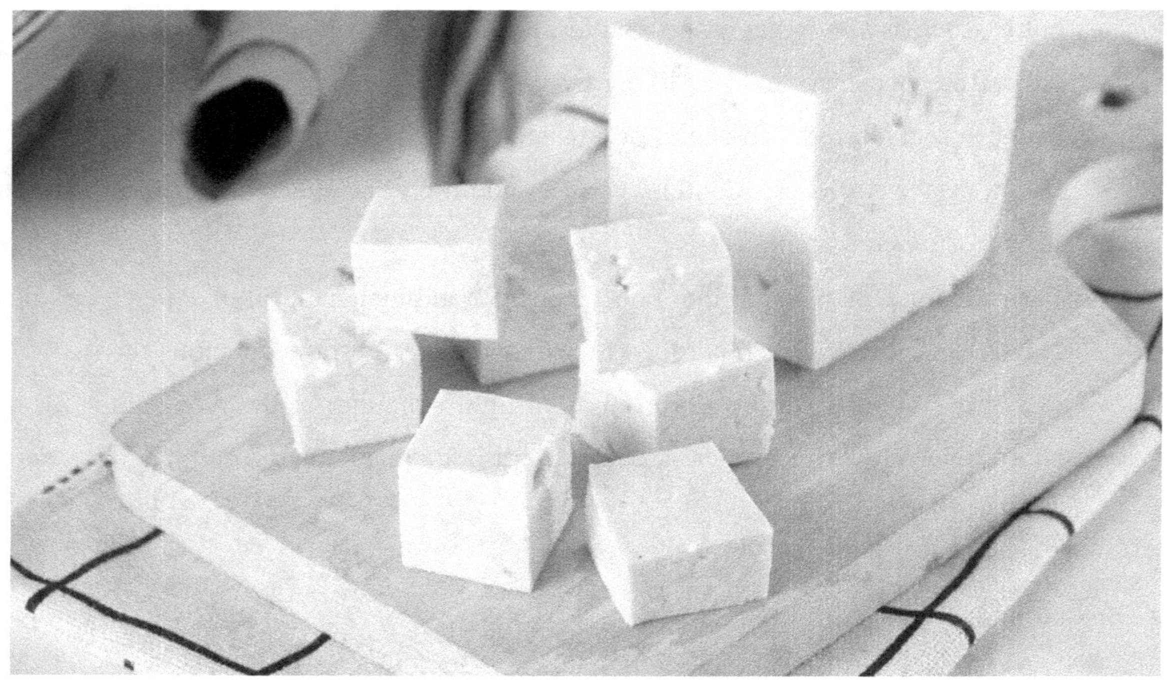

Chipotle Tofu Chilaquiles redefines brunch. Crispy tortilla chips meet smoky chipotle-marinated tofu, topped with zesty salsa and avocado. This plant-based twist on a traditional dish offers a medley of textures and flavors—a spicy, savory delight that's both hearty and satisfying.

Preparation Time: 10 minutes

Cook Time: 35 minutes

Total Time: 45 minutes

Serves: 2

Difficulty: Medium

Ingredients:

- 200g of tofu, pressed and diced
- 1 chipotle pepper in adobo sauce, minced
- 1 tablespoon of olive oil
- 1 small onion, diced
- 2 cloves of garlic, minced
- 1 red bell pepper, diced
- 1 can (400g) of diced tomatoes
- 1 teaspoon of ground cumin
- 1/2 teaspoon of smoked paprika
- Salt and pepper, to taste
- 12 small corn tortillas, cut into triangles
- 1 cup of vegan cheese, shredded
- 1 avocado, diced
- Fresh cilantro, chopped, for garnish

Kitchen Tools Needed:

- Saucepan
- Baking sheet
- Skillet

xxxxxxxxxxxxxxxxxxxx

Instructions:

a. Preheat your oven to 180°C (350°F).

b. In a saucepan, warm the olive oil over medium heat. Add the diced tofu and cook until it turns golden brown. Once done, remove the tofu from the saucepan and set it aside.

c. In the same saucepan, add the minced chipotle pepper, onion, garlic, and red bell pepper. Sauté them until the vegetables become tender.

d. Incorporate the diced tomatoes, ground cumin, smoked paprika, salt, and pepper into the mixture. Stir well to ensure all the flavors meld together, and let it simmer for approximately 5 minutes.

e. While the sauce simmers, place the tortilla triangles on a baking sheet and bake for about 10 minutes or until they become crispy.

f. In a skillet, arrange a layer of the baked tortilla triangles. Top this layer with half of the cooked vegetables, tofu, and vegan cheese. Then, repeat these layers once more.

g. Cover the skillet and cook over low heat for 5 minutes or until the vegan cheese has melted beautifully.

h. To serve, garnish your Chipotle Tofu Chilaquiles with diced avocado and fresh cilantro.

Cooking Notes:

- Customize your chilaquiles by adding extras like black beans, corn, or jalapeños for more flavor and texture.
- Adjust the level of spiciness by varying the amount of chipotle pepper used in the recipe. Be cautious, as chipotle can be quite hot.
- To make the dish even heartier, consider topping it with a dollop of vegan sour cream or a drizzle of hot sauce.
- Chilaquiles are often enjoyed for breakfast or brunch, but they make a satisfying meal any time of day.
- Feel free to experiment with different vegan cheeses to find your favorite flavor combination.

13. Fluffy Chickpea Scramble

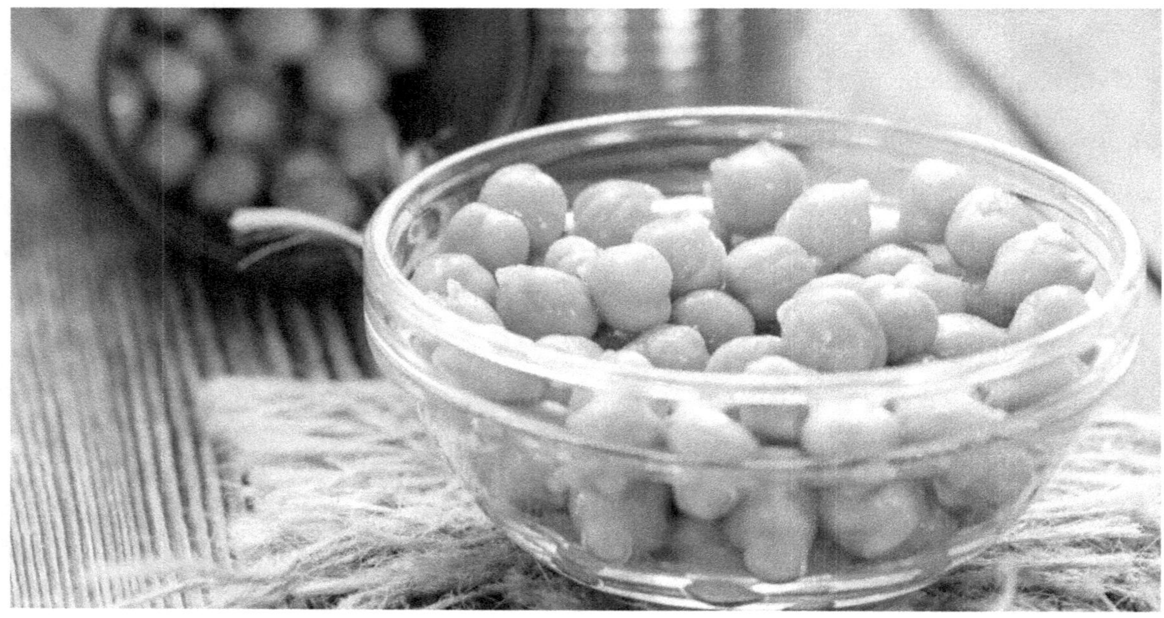

Fluffy Chickpea Scramble elevates breakfast. Whipped chickpea batter, seasoned with herbs and spices, creates a satisfying and protein-rich alternative to traditional scrambled eggs. This plant-based creation offers a creamy texture and savory taste, making for a flavorful and nutritious start to the day.

Preparation Time: 10 minutes

Cook Time: 35 minutes

Total Time: 45 minutes

Serves: 2

Difficulty: Medium

Ingredients:

- 1 cup of canned chickpeas
- 1 tablespoon of olive oil
- 1 small onion, diced
- 1 bell pepper, diced
- 2 cloves of garlic, minced
- 1 teaspoon of turmeric
- 1/2 teaspoon of cumin
- 1/4 teaspoon of paprika
- Salt and pepper to taste
- 2 tablespoons of nutritional yeast
- 2 tablespoons of chopped fresh parsley
- 2 tablespoons of chopped green onions

Kitchen Tools Needed:

- Stovetop
- Non-stick pan
- Spatula
- Bowl

xxxxxxxxxxxxxxxxxxx

Instructions:

a. Start by draining and rinsing the canned chickpeas.

b. Heat up some olive oil in a non-stick skillet over medium heat.

c. Add in the diced onion, bell pepper, and minced garlic to the skillet. Sauté them for about 4-5 minutes until they become soft and tender.

d. Introduce the drained chickpeas to the skillet and give them a light mash using a fork or a potato masher.

e. Stir in the turmeric, cumin, paprika, salt, and pepper, ensuring that all the spices blend well.

f. Continue cooking for another 5-6 minutes, occasionally stirring, until the chickpeas are heated through and have developed a slight crispiness.

g. Remove the skillet from the heat and generously sprinkle nutritional yeast, chopped parsley, and green onions over the chickpea mixture.

h. Serve the fluffy chickpea scramble while it's still warm and savor the flavors!

Cooking Notes:

- You can customize your chickpea scramble by adding your favorite veggies like spinach, tomatoes, or mushrooms.
- Don't shy away from experimenting with different spices and seasonings to suit your taste.
- This scramble is a versatile dish; enjoy it on its own, as a filling for sandwiches, or even as a topping for salads.
- For a creamier texture, consider adding a splash of plant-based milk while sautéing the chickpeas.
- This recipe is perfect for breakfast, brunch, or a quick dinner.

14. Roasted Sweet Potato & Kale Breakfast Hash

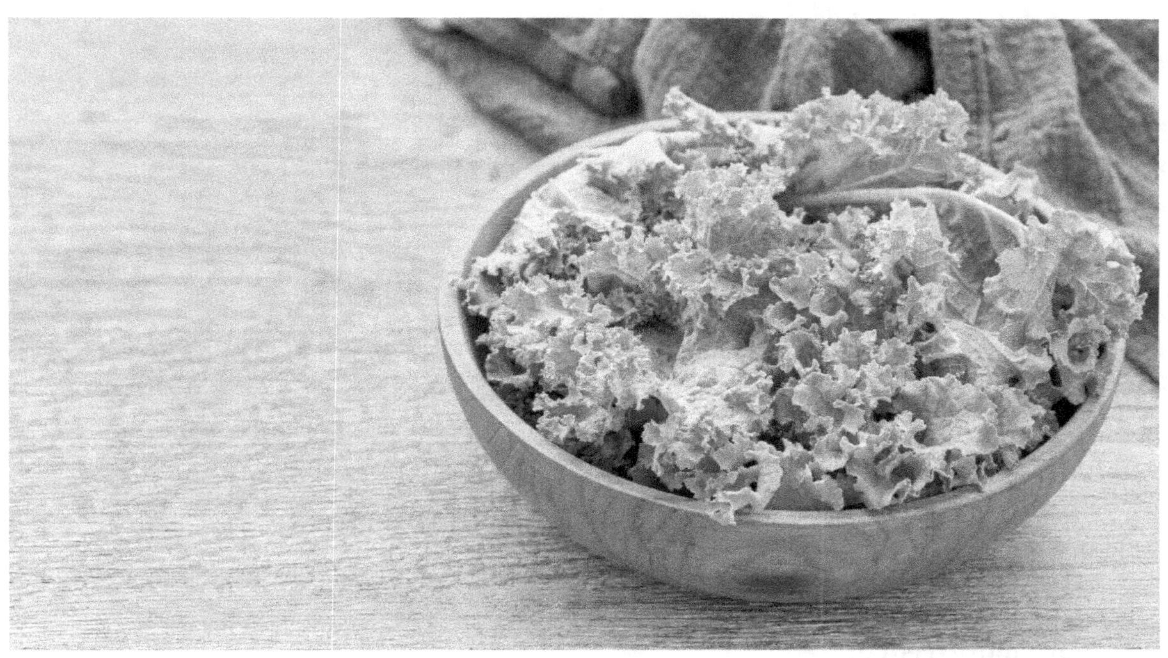

Roasted Sweet Potato & Kale Breakfast Hash redefines mornings. A medley of sweet potatoes, hearty kale, and savory spices creates a flavorful, nutrient-packed dish. This satisfying and colorful breakfast offers a wholesome start to the day that's both delicious and nourishing.

Preparation Time: 10 minutes

Cook Time: 35 minutes

Total Time: 45 minutes

Serves: 2

Difficulty: Medium

Ingredients:

- 2 medium sweet potatoes, cubed
- 2 cups of chopped kale
- 1 small red onion, thinly sliced
- 2 cloves of garlic, minced
- 1 tablespoon of olive oil
- Salt and pepper to taste
- 1 teaspoon of paprika
- 1/2 teaspoon of ground cumin
- 1/4 teaspoon of chili flakes
- 2 tablespoons of nutritional yeast
- 1 avocado, sliced
- 1 tablespoon of fresh parsley, chopped

Kitchen Tools Needed:

- oven
- skillet

XXXXXXXXXXXXXXXXXXX

Instructions:

a. Preheat your oven to 425°F (220°C).

b. Take the cubed sweet potatoes and spread them out on a baking sheet. Drizzle some olive oil over them and give them a good toss to make sure they're evenly coated. Season with salt, pepper, paprika, and ground cumin.

c. Roast those beautifully seasoned sweet potatoes in the preheated oven for about 20-25 minutes until they turn a lovely golden color and get wonderfully crispy.

d. Meanwhile, in a skillet, warm some olive oil over medium heat. Add the sliced onion and minced garlic, sautéing until the onion becomes translucent and you can smell the fragrant garlic.

e. Toss the chopped kale into the skillet and cook until it wilts down nicely.

f. Season the mixture with salt, pepper, and a pinch of chili flakes for some extra zing.

g. Once your sweet potatoes are done roasting, introduce them to the pan with the vibrant greens. Give everything a good toss to mix it up beautifully.

h. Now, sprinkle some nutritional yeast over the mixture and gently toss again to make sure it's well coated.

i. Take the pan off the heat, and split the hash onto two plates.

j. Finish it off with slices of creamy avocado and a sprinkle of freshly chopped parsley.

k. Voilà! Your Roasted Sweet Potato & Kale Breakfast Hash is ready to be savored.

Cooking Notes:

- Feel free to customize your hash with extras like shredded cheese, a poached or fried egg on top, or a drizzle of hot sauce for some added flair.
- This hash is versatile – it works just as well for brunch or lunch as it does for breakfast.
- Try different seasoning combinations to suit your taste buds. Smoked paprika, rosemary, or thyme are great options.
- Make sure to cut the sweet potatoes into evenly sized cubes so they cook uniformly.
- Keep an eye on the kale; it can go from wilted to overcooked fairly quickly, so it's best to sauté it just until it's tender.

15. Masala–Spiced Tofu Scramble

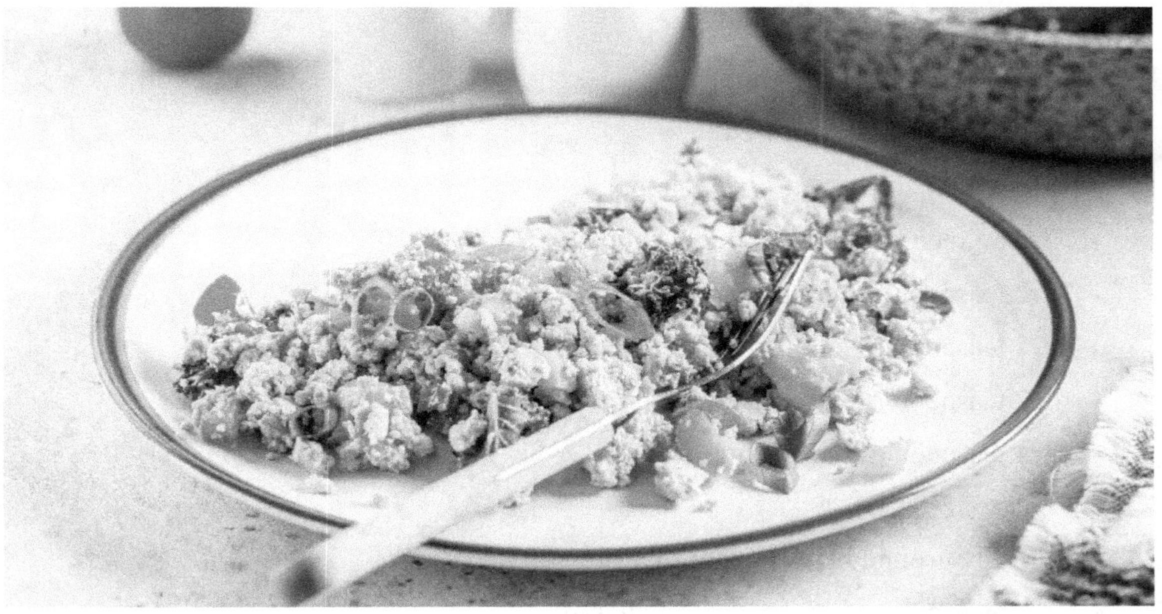

Masala-Spiced Tofu Scramble adds a bold twist to breakfast. Tofu, infused with aromatic masala spices, creates a protein-packed scramble. This flavorful and hearty plant-based option offers a touch of Indian-inspired warmth and a satisfying start to the day with a burst of savory flavors.

Preparation Time: 10 minutes

Cook Time: 35 minutes

Total Time: 45 minutes

Serves: 2

Difficulty: Medium

Ingredients:

- 200g tofu
- 1 tablespoon of olive oil
- 1 small onion, finely chopped
- 2 cloves of garlic, minced
- 1/2 a red bell pepper, finely chopped
- 1/2 a green bell pepper, finely chopped
- 1/2 teaspoon of turmeric powder
- 1/2 teaspoon of cumin powder
- 1/2 teaspoon of coriander powder
- 1/4 teaspoon of chili powder
- Salt to taste
- Freshly ground black pepper to taste
- 2 tablespoons of chopped fresh cilantro
- 2 slices of bread, toasted

Kitchen Tools Needed:

- skillet
- spatula

XXXXXXXXXXXXXXXXXXXX

Instructions:

a. Start by heating up some olive oil in a skillet over medium heat.

b. Throw in the chopped onion and garlic. Let them sizzle away until they turn that beautiful translucent color.

c. Now, crumble your tofu right into the skillet. Cook it for about 5 minutes, giving it a stir now and then.

d. It's bell pepper time! Add the chopped peppers and let them join the flavorful party for another 3 minutes.

e. Get ready to spice things up. Sprinkle in the turmeric powder, coriander powder, cumin powder, chili powder, salt, and black pepper. Make sure everything gets a good coating of those aromatic spices.

f. Cook it all up for an extra 2 minutes or until the tofu warms through and those spices work their magic.

g. Take your skillet off the heat and sprinkle a generous helping of freshly chopped cilantro over the tofu scramble.

h. It's time to plate up! Spoon that delicious tofu scramble onto some slices of toasted bread.

i. Serve it up piping hot, and get ready to enjoy a flavorful breakfast!

Cooking Notes:

- Customize your spice level by adjusting the amount of chili powder. More for the heat lovers, less for those who prefer milder flavors.

- Don't shy away from experimenting with your favorite veggies. Mushrooms, spinach, or tomatoes can all be fantastic additions.

- Feel free to serve this scramble with other sides like avocado slices, salsa, or a dollop of yogurt for added richness.

16. Baked Sweet Potatoes 2 Ways!

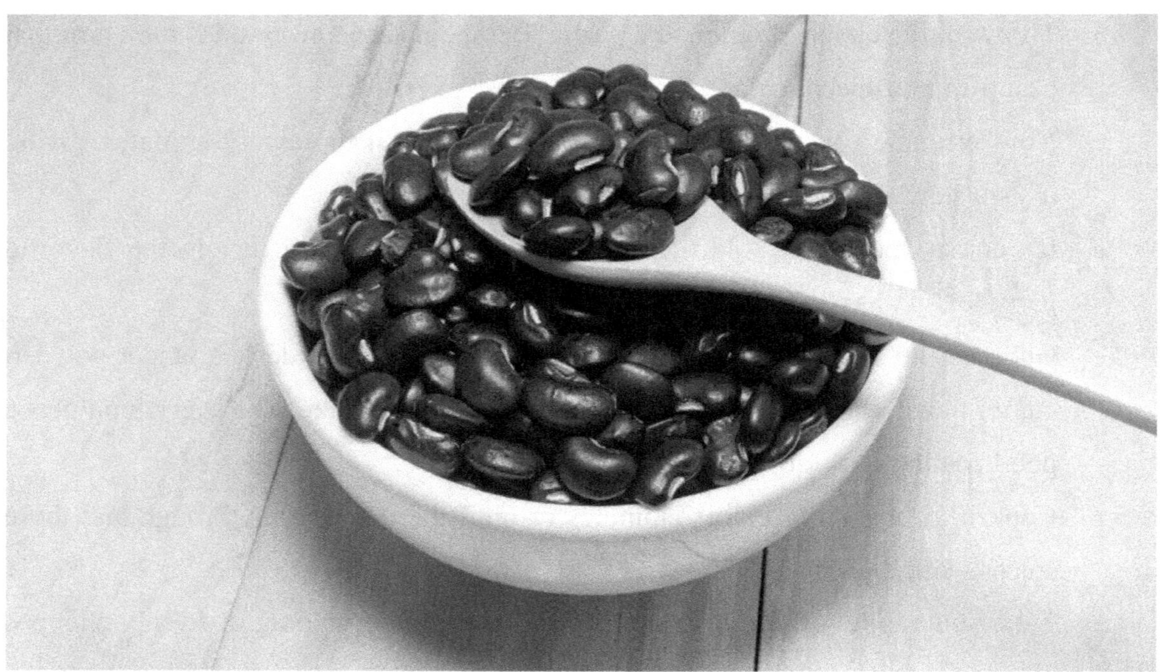

Baked Sweet Potatoes 2 Ways is a versatile delight. One half is adorned with savory toppings—beans, herbs—creating a hearty and balanced option. The other half gets a sweet treatment with cinnamon and nut butter. This colorful dish offers a dual journey of flavors in a single plate.

Preparation Time: 10 minutes

Cook Time: 35 minutes

Total Time: 45 minutes

Serves: 1

Difficulty: Medium

Ingredients:

- 1 medium-sized sweet potato
- 1 tablespoon of olive oil
- Salt and pepper to taste
- For Sweet Option:
- 1 tablespoon of maple syrup
- 1/4 teaspoon of cinnamon

For Savory Option:

- 1/4 cup of black beans
- 1/4 cup of salsa
- 1/4 of an avocado, sliced

Kitchen Tools Needed:

- Oven
- Baking sheet
- Knife

XXXXXXXXXXXXXXXXXXX

Instructions:

a. Preheat your oven to 400°F (200°C).

b. Begin by thoroughly washing and scrubbing the sweet potatoes.

c. To ensure even cooking, gently puncture the sweet potatoes with a fork in a few places.

d. Now, take each sweet potato and generously rub it with olive oil, and then season with a pinch of salt and pepper.

e. Place the prepared sweet potatoes on a baking sheet and proceed to bake them for approximately 30-35 minutes or until they become tender.

Sweet Option:

a. In a small bowl, combine a delightful mixture of maple syrup and cinnamon.

b. Once the sweet potatoes are done baking, remove them from the oven and drizzle this sweet concoction over them.

Savory Option:

a. For a savory twist, top the baked sweet potatoes with a flavorful combination of black beans, salsa, and sliced avocado.

b. Serve up your delicious creations and savor the wonderful flavors!

Cooking Notes:

- Sweet potatoes vary in size, so adjust the baking time accordingly. Larger ones may take a bit longer to become tender.
- Ensure even cooking by selecting sweet potatoes of similar sizes.
- Feel free to customize your toppings to suit your taste. You can add cheese, sour cream, or other favorite toppings to enhance the flavor.
- Don't forget to let the sweet potatoes cool for a few minutes before adding toppings or serving to avoid burning yourself.
- These baked sweet potatoes are a versatile side dish or even a main course. Experiment with different toppings and seasonings to suit your preferences.

17. Cheesy Broccoli Hashbrown Bake (Oil-Free)

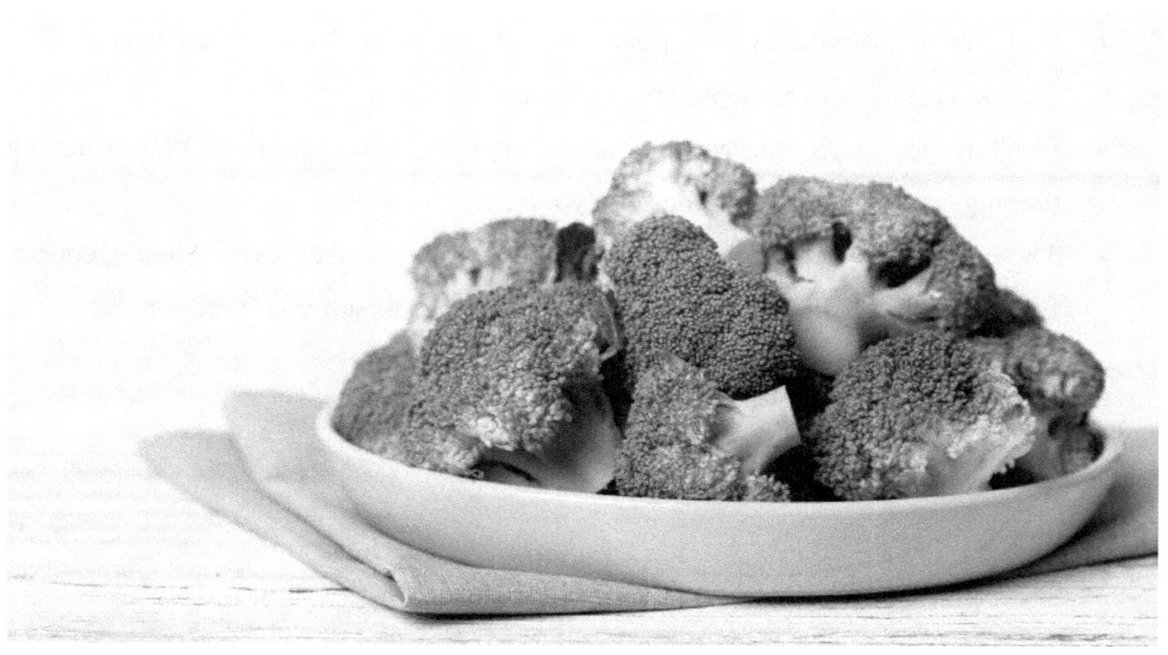

Cheesy Broccoli Hashbrown Bake (Oil-Free) is a guilt-free indulgence. Crispy shredded potatoes meet tender broccoli, enveloped in a creamy, dairy-free cheese sauce. This wholesome and flavorful dish offers a savory experience with a touch of comfort, celebrating both taste and healthfulness in each bite.

Preparation Time: 10 minutes

Cook Time: 55 minutes

Total Time: 1 hour 5 minutes

Serves: 6

Difficulty: Medium

Ingredients:

- 800g of frozen hashbrowns
- 400g of broccoli florets
- 1 onion, diced
- 4 cloves of garlic, minced
- 2 cups of plant-based cheese, shredded
- 1 cup of unsweetened plant-based milk
- 1/4 cup of nutritional yeast
- 2 tablespoons of cornstarch
- 1 tablespoon of tamari or soy sauce
- 1/2 teaspoon of smoked paprika
- 1/2 teaspoon of dried thyme
- 1/2 teaspoon of salt
- 1/4 teaspoon of black pepper

Kitchen Tools Needed:

- Oven
- Baking sheet
- Knife

XXXXXXXXXXXXXXXXXXX

Instructions:

a. Start by preheating your oven to 375°F (190°C).

b. In a large bowl, combine the following ingredients: frozen hashbrowns, broccoli florets, diced onion, minced garlic, shredded plant-based cheese, plant-based milk, nutritional yeast, cornstarch, tamari or soy sauce, smoked paprika, dried thyme, salt, and black pepper. Be sure to mix everything together thoroughly.

c. Transfer the well-mixed mixture into a greased 9x13-inch baking dish.

d. Place the baking dish into the preheated oven and bake for approximately 40-45 minutes, or until the top becomes delightfully golden brown and crispy.

e. Once done, take it out of the oven and allow it to cool for a few minutes before serving.

f. Serve this delightful Cheesy Broccoli Hashbrown Bake while it's warm and savor the flavors!

Cooking Notes:

- You can easily customize this dish by adding other vegetables or spices that you prefer, making it your own unique creation.
- Ensure the hashbrowns are thawed before mixing them into the recipe for even cooking.
- Leftovers can be refrigerated and reheated for a quick and delicious meal the next day.
- Feel free to experiment with different plant-based cheeses to find your favorite flavor combination.
- For a hint of freshness, garnish with chopped herbs like parsley or chives before serving.

18. Sweet Potato with Black Bean Dip

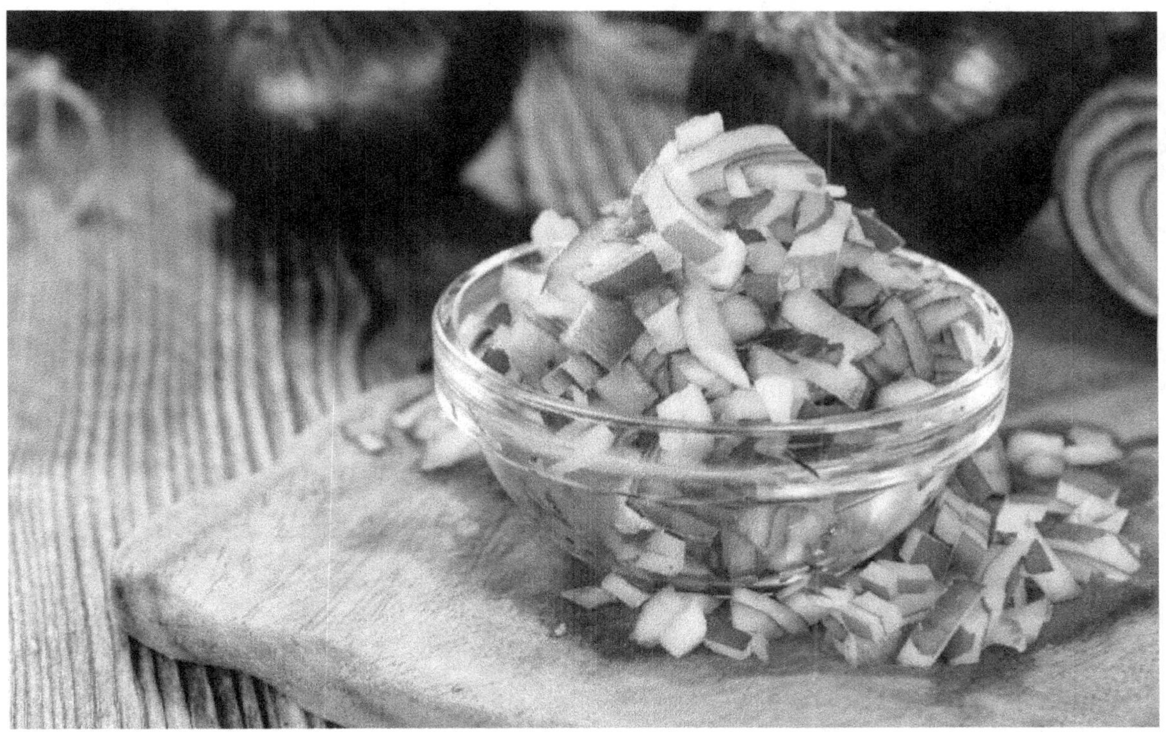

Sweet Potato with Black Bean Dip brings a kick to snacking. Roasted sweet potatoes and black beans meet zesty spices, creating a flavorful and nutritious dip. With a hint of smokiness, it's a versatile option that adds a Southwestern flair to chips, veggies, or wraps—a bold and wholesome treat.

Preparation Time: 10 minutes

Cook Time: 55 minutes

Total Time: 1 hour 5 minutes

Serves: 6

Difficulty: Medium

Ingredients:

- 2 large, sweet potatoes, peeled and diced
- 1 can (15 oz) of black beans, drained and rinsed
- 1/2 cup of diced red onion
- 1/2 cup of diced red bell pepper
- 1 jalapeno, seeded and diced
- 2 cloves of garlic, minced
- 1/4 cup of fresh lime juice
- 1/4 cup of chopped fresh cilantro
- 1 teaspoon of ground cumin
- 1/2 teaspoon of chili powder
- Salt and pepper, to taste

Kitchen Tools Needed:

- Baking sheet
- Blender
- Mixing bowl

XXXXXXXXXXXXXXXXXXXX

Instructions:

a. Preheat your oven to 400°F (200°C).

b. Spread the diced sweet potatoes evenly on a baking sheet and roast them for approximately 25-30 minutes, or until they become tender.

c. In a blender, combine the roasted sweet potatoes with black beans, red onion, red bell pepper, jalapeno, garlic, lime juice, cilantro, cumin, chili powder, salt, and pepper.

d. Blend the mixture until it reaches a smooth and creamy consistency.

e. Transfer the dip from the blender into a mixing bowl, then refrigerate it for a minimum of 15 minutes to allow the flavors to blend harmoniously.

f. Serve this delightful Southwest Sweet Potato Black Bean Dip with tortilla chips or sliced vegetables.

g. Savor the flavors and enjoy!

Cooking Notes:

- Adjust the spice level by modifying the amount of jalapeno used, depending on your heat preference.
- This dip can be prepared in advance and refrigerated for even more robust flavor.
- Experiment with different dippers like pita bread, crackers, or even as a sandwich spread for a variety of serving options.
- Customize the dip by adding toppings like diced avocado, shredded cheese, or a dollop of sour cream for an extra layer of indulgence.
- Leftovers can be stored in an airtight container in the refrigerator for a couple of days, making it a convenient snack or appetizer for later enjoyment.

19. Collard Green Wraps with Green Curry Tahini Sauce

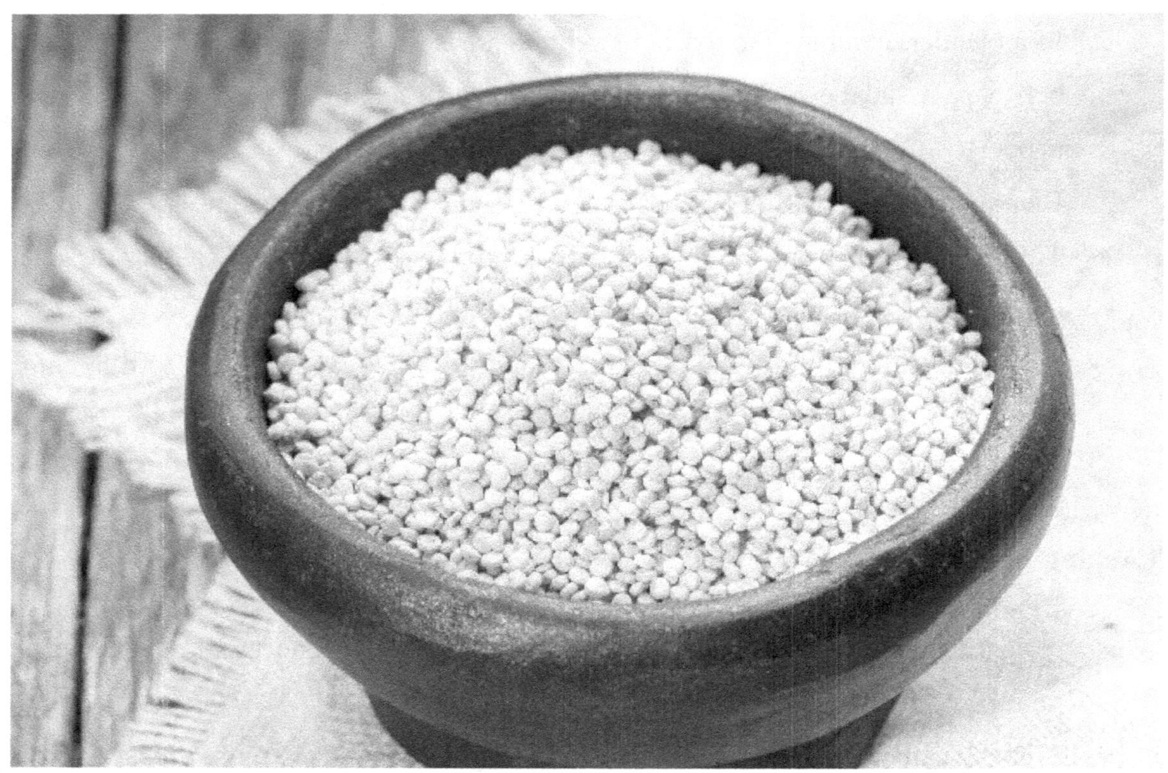

Collard Green Wraps with Green Curry Tahini Sauce offer a rainbow of flavors. Collard greens envelop colorful veggies, avocado, and quinoa, drizzled with zesty green curry tahini sauce. This plant-powered creation delivers a harmonious blend of textures and tastes, celebrating health and vibrancy in each bite.

Preparation Time: 10 minutes

Cook Time: 55 minutes

Total Time: 1 hour 5 minutes

Serves: 6

Difficulty: Medium

Ingredients:

- 4 large collard green leaves
- 1 cup of cooked quinoa
- 1 cup of shredded carrots
- 1 cup of thinly sliced cucumbers
- 1/2 cup of thinly sliced red bell peppers
- 1/2 cup of fresh cilantro leaves
- 1/4 cup of chopped roasted peanuts

For the green curry tahini sauce:

- 1/4 cup of tahini
- 2 tablespoons of lime juice
- 2 tablespoons of soy sauce
- 1 tablespoon of maple syrup
- 1 tablespoon of green curry paste
- 1 clove of garlic
- 1/4 cup of water

Kitchen Tools Needed:

- Knife
- Cutting Board
- Blender
- Bowl

xxxxxxxxxxxxxxxxxxx

Instructions:

a. Begin by preparing the collard green leaves. Remove the stems and blanch them in boiling water for 1 minute, then drain and set them aside.

b. In a blender, combine all the ingredients required for the green curry tahini sauce and blend until you achieve a smooth consistency. Set this sauce aside.

c. Lay out a collard green leaf on a flat surface and place a portion of cooked quinoa onto the leaf, leaving about 1 inch of space at the top.

d. Top the quinoa with shredded carrots, sliced cucumbers, red bell peppers, cilantro leaves, and chopped peanuts.

e. Drizzle a generous amount of the green curry tahini sauce over the filling.

f. Roll the collard green leaf tightly, tucking in the sides as you roll.

g. Repeat this process with the remaining collard green leaves and filling ingredients.

h. Once you've prepared all the wraps, carefully slice each one in half and get ready to serve.

i. Finally, savor the vibrant flavors of your collard green wraps with green curry tahini sauce!

Cooking Notes:

- To make these wraps more substantial, consider adding protein sources like grilled chicken, tofu, or chickpeas to the filling.
- Customize the fillings with your favorite vegetables or herbs to suit your taste preferences.
- Collard green leaves are a sturdy choice for wraps, but you can also use other large leafy greens like Swiss chard or lettuce if preferred.
- If you prefer a spicier sauce, increase the amount of green curry paste or add a dash of hot sauce to the tahini mixture.
- These wraps are perfect for meal prep, as they can be assembled in advance and enjoyed throughout the week. Just store the sauce separately to keep the wraps fresh.

20. Kale Falafel Hummus Wraps

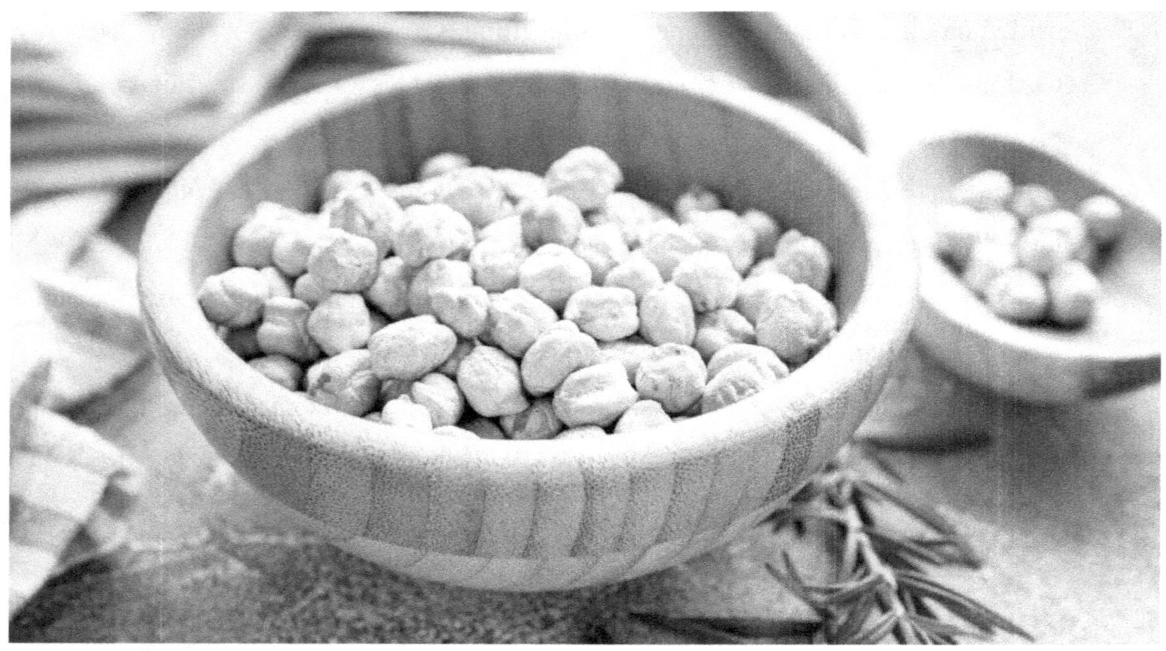

Kale Falafel Hummus Wraps redefine wrap perfection. Crispy kale-falafel balls join creamy hummus, fresh veggies, and tangy sauces, all enveloped in a soft tortilla. This plant-based delight offers a medley of textures and flavors, creating a satisfying and nutritious handheld feast.

Preparation Time: 10 minutes

Cook Time: 55 minutes

Total Time: 1 hour 5 minutes

Serves: 4

Difficulty: Medium

Ingredients:

- 200g of kale
- 1 can of chickpeas, drained
- 2 cloves of garlic
- 1/2 cup of breadcrumbs
- 1/4 cup of chopped parsley
- 1/4 cup of chopped cilantro
- 1 teaspoon of cumin
- 1 teaspoon of coriander
- 1/2 teaspoon of salt
- 1/4 teaspoon of black pepper
- 4 tablespoons of tahini
- 4 large tortillas
- 1 cup of shredded carrots
- 1 cup of sliced cucumber
- 1 cup of cherry tomatoes, halved
- 1/2 cup of red onion, thinly sliced

Kitchen Tools Needed:

- oven
- food processor
- baking sheet
- knife
- cutting board
- mixing bowl
- measuring cups

Instructions:

a. Start by preheating your oven to 400°F (200°C).

b. In a food processor, combine kale, chickpeas, garlic, breadcrumbs, parsley, cilantro, cumin, coriander, salt, and black pepper. Process until the mixture is well combined.

c. Shape the mixture into small falafel patties and arrange them on a greased baking sheet.

d. Bake the falafels for 20-25 minutes or until they turn a beautiful golden brown and become crispy.

e. While the falafels are in the oven, prepare the hummus by mixing tahini with 2 tablespoons of water in a mixing bowl. Stir until you achieve a smooth and creamy consistency.

f. To assemble the wraps, generously spread hummus on each tortilla.

g. Place a few falafel patties on top of the hummus.

h. Add a handful of shredded carrots, cucumber slices, cherry tomatoes, and red onion slices onto the falafels.

i. Roll up the tortillas tightly and then slice them in half for serving.

j. If desired, serve the kale falafel hummus wraps with extra hummus on the side.

Cooking Notes:

- Feel free to customize your wraps by adding your favorite vegetables or sauces to suit your taste preferences.
- These wraps can be made in advance for a quick and convenient lunch or dinner option.
- For extra flavor, you can drizzle some olive oil and a squeeze of lemon juice over the assembled wraps before rolling them up.
- If you want a spicier kick, consider adding hot sauce or Sriracha to the hummus or as a condiment.
- These wraps are a great way to incorporate more greens into your diet, and you can experiment with different types of greens, like spinach or arugula, if preferred.

21. Curried Quinoa Chickpea Burgers

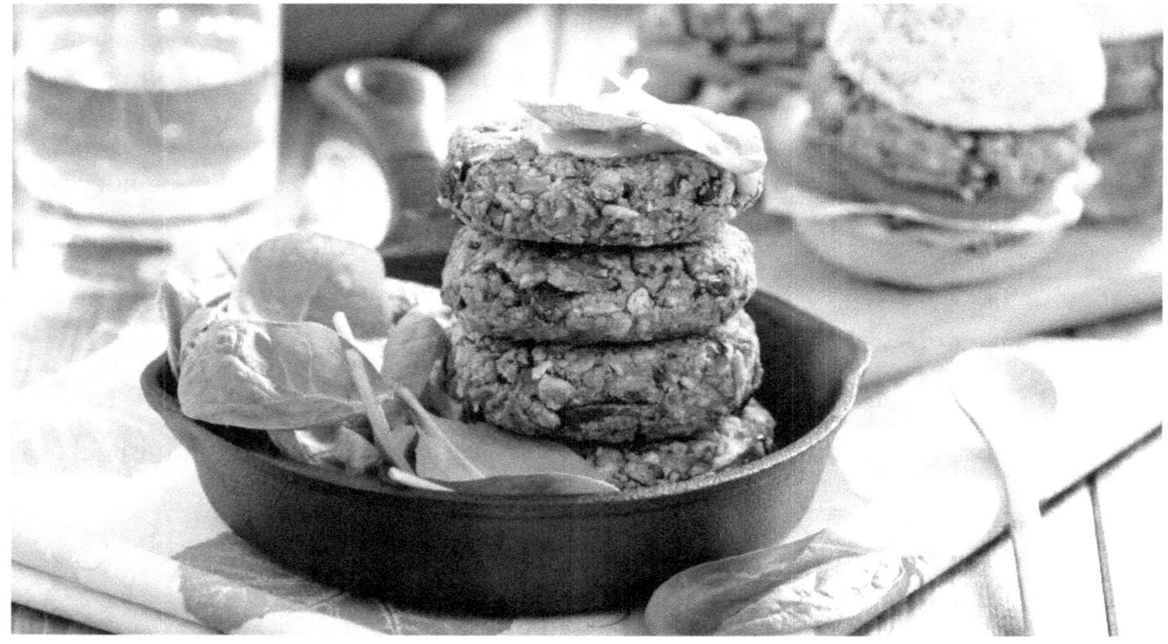

Curried Quinoa Chickpea Burgers bring global fusion. Nutty quinoa, chickpeas, and aromatic curry spices come together, forming hearty patties. Topped with vibrant veggies and sauces, they offer a flavorful and protein-packed alternative to traditional burgers—a wholesome and tasty culinary adventure in every bite.

Preparation Time: 10 minutes

Cook Time: 55 minutes

Total Time: 1 hour 5 minutes

Serves: 4

Difficulty: Medium

Ingredients:

- 1 cup of cooked quinoa
- 1 can of chickpeas, drained and rinsed
- 1/4 cup of breadcrumbs
- 1/4 cup of finely chopped onion
- 2 cloves of garlic, minced
- 1 teaspoon of curry powder
- 1/2 teaspoon of cumin
- 1/4 teaspoon of paprika
- Salt and pepper to taste
- 4 burger buns
- Lettuce, tomato, and onion for garnish

Kitchen Tools Needed:

- Mixing bowl
- Food processor
- Frying pan
- Spatula

XXXXXXXXXXXXXXXXXXXX

Instructions:

a. Begin by mashing the chickpeas in a mixing bowl, using either a fork or a food processor.

b. To the mashed chickpeas, add cooked breadcrumbs, quinoa, finely chopped onion, minced garlic, curry powder, cumin, paprika, salt, and pepper. Ensure thorough mixing until all ingredients are well combined.

c. Divide the mixture into 4 equal portions and shape each portion into a patty.

d. In a frying pan over medium heat, melt a drizzle of oil. Cook the patties for about 4-5 minutes per side, or until they achieve a beautiful golden brown and crisp texture.

e. If desired, toast the burger buns.

f. Assemble your burgers by placing a patty on each bun and topping them with lettuce, tomato, and onion.

g. Serve your Curried Quinoa Chickpea Burgers along with your preferred sauce or condiments.

Cooking Notes:

- Customize your burger toppings with additional ingredients like avocado slices, pickles, or cheese to suit your taste preferences.
- These burgers can also be cooked on a grill for a smoky flavor and attractive grill marks.
- For a gluten-free option, use gluten-free breadcrumbs and buns.
- Consider adding a yogurt-based cucumber sauce or tzatziki for a refreshing and tangy flavor element.
- Leftover patties can be refrigerated and enjoyed later or crumbled into salads or wraps for added protein and flavor.
- These burgers are a great meatless option for vegetarians and can be made vegan by using egg replacers like flax eggs or chickpea flour as a binding agent.

22. Smoky BBQ Black Bean Burger

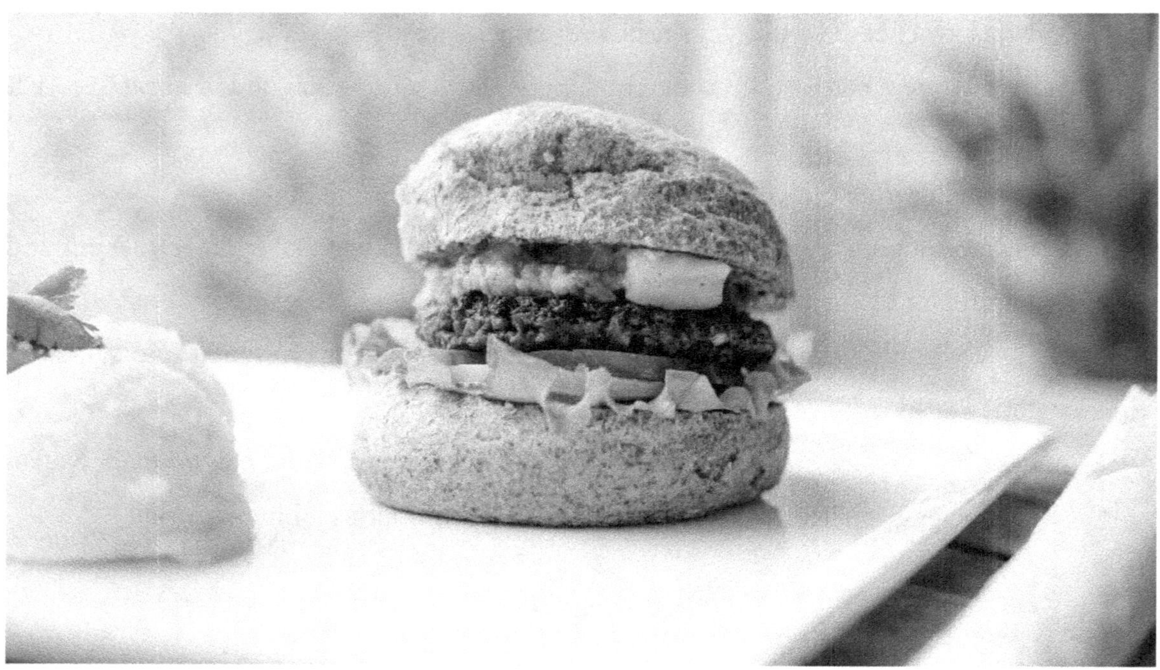

Smoky BBQ Black Bean Burger is a grill-worthy delight. Flavorful black bean patty, kissed with smoky barbecue sauce, takes center stage. Layered with crunchy veggies and served on a bun, it's a plant-based twist on a classic that delivers a satisfying combination of tastes and textures.

Preparation Time: 10 minutes

Cook Time: 55 minutes

Total Time: 1 hour 5 minutes

Serves: 4

Difficulty: Medium

Ingredients:

- 1 can (15 ounces) of black beans, drained and rinsed
- 1/2 cup of breadcrumbs
- 1/4 cup of finely chopped onion
- 2 cloves of garlic, minced
- 2 tablespoons of tomato paste
- 1 tablespoon of soy sauce
- 1 teaspoon of smoked paprika
- 1/2 teaspoon of cumin
- 1/4 teaspoon of cayenne pepper
- Salt and pepper to taste
- 4 burger buns
- Toppings of your choice (lettuce, tomato, onion, avocado, etc.)

Kitchen Tools Needed:

- grill
- food processor
- mixing bowl

xxxxxxxxxxxxxxxxxxxx

Instructions:

a. Start by using a food processor to combine black beans, breadcrumbs, onion, garlic, tomato paste, soy sauce, smoked paprika, cumin, cayenne pepper, salt, and pepper. Pulse the mixture until it's well combined and slightly chunky.

b. Shape this mixture into 4 patties and place them on a baking sheet lined with parchment paper. Refrigerate them for 30 minutes to help them firm up.

c. Preheat your grill to medium heat and lightly oil the grill grates.

d. Grill the patties for approximately 4-5 minutes per side, or until they are heated through and display those enticing grill marks.

e. If desired, you can toast the burger buns on the grill for about a minute.

f. Assemble your burgers by placing one patty on each bun and topping them with your preferred ingredients.

Cooking Notes:

- Customize your toppings with favorites like lettuce, tomato, cheese, pickles, or barbecue sauce.

- For a vegan version, consider using egg substitutes like flax eggs or chickpea flour as binding agents.

- Experiment with different beans like kidney beans or chickpeas for unique flavors and textures.

- To prevent burgers from sticking to the grill, make sure they are well-chilled before grilling.

- If grilling isn't an option, you can also cook these burgers on a stovetop grill pan or in the oven. Adjust cooking times accordingly.

23. Raw Rainbow Veggie Noodle Salad with Peanut Dressing

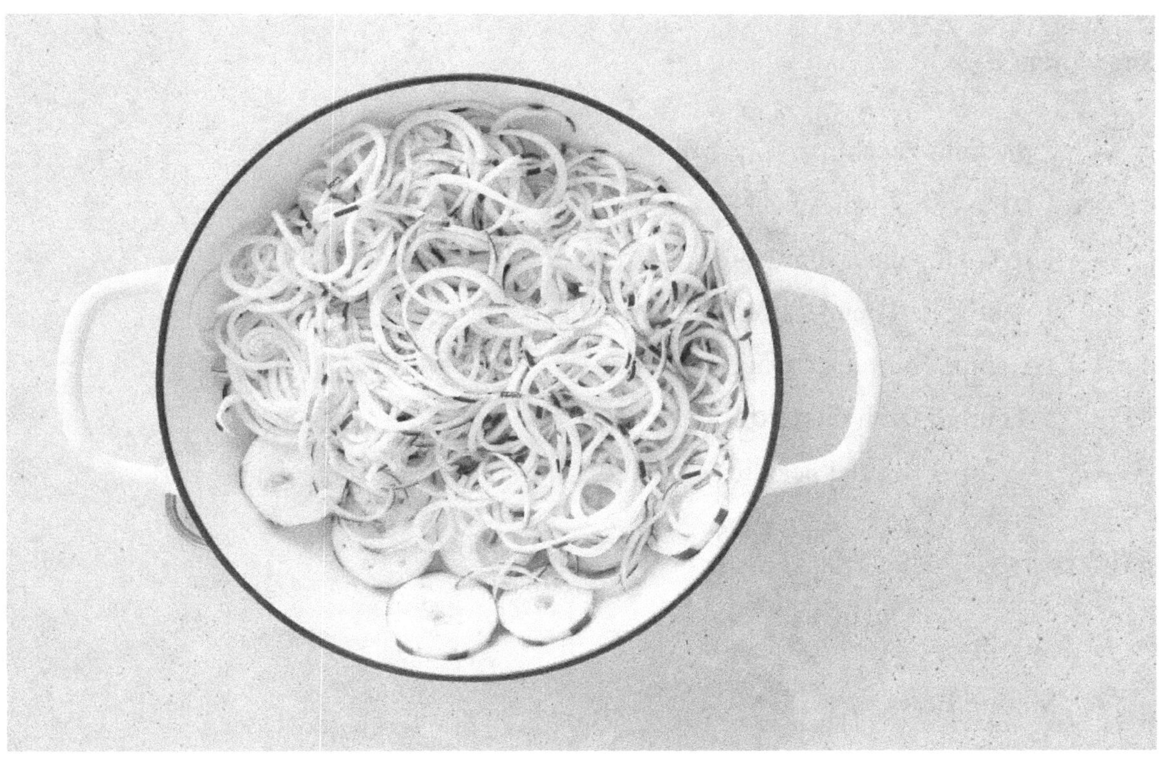

Raw Rainbow Veggie Noodle Salad with Peanut Dressing is a vibrant feast. Colorful spiralized veggies meet a creamy peanut dressing, creating a refreshing and healthful dish. With a burst of colors, textures, and flavors, it's a celebration of freshness and wholesomeness in a single bowl.

Preparation Time: 10 minutes

Cook Time: 55 minutes

Total Time: 1 hour 5 minutes

Serves:2

Difficulty: Medium

Ingredients:

- 2 medium zucchinis, spiralized
- 1 large carrot, spiralized
- 1 red bell pepper, thinly sliced
- 1 yellow bell pepper, thinly sliced
- 1/2 cup of purple cabbage, shredded
- 1/4 cup of fresh cilantro, chopped
- 1/4 cup of roasted peanuts, chopped

Kitchen Tools Needed:

- Spiralizer
- Mixing Bowl
- Whisk

xxxxxxxxxxxxxxxxxxx

Instructions:

a. Begin by whisking together the peanut dressing ingredients in a mixing bowl until they are well combined.

b. Add the spiralized zucchinis, carrot, red bell pepper, yellow bell pepper, and purple cabbage to the bowl.

c. Toss the vegetables with the peanut dressing to ensure they are evenly coated.

d. Finish by sprinkling chopped cilantro and roasted peanuts over the salad.

e. You can serve it right away or refrigerate it until you're ready to enjoy.

Cooking Notes:

- Feel free to customize the vegetables in this salad based on your preferences or what's in season.
- Add grilled chicken, tofu, or shrimp for a protein boost if desired.
- If you like it spicy, consider adding a pinch of red pepper flakes to the dressing for some heat.
- This salad is perfect for meal prep as it stays fresh in the refrigerator for a few days.
- Experiment with different nut options like cashews or almonds for added crunch and flavor.
- Adjust the consistency of the dressing by adding a bit more water or lime juice if needed.

24. Grilled Romaine Caesar Salad with Herbed White Beans

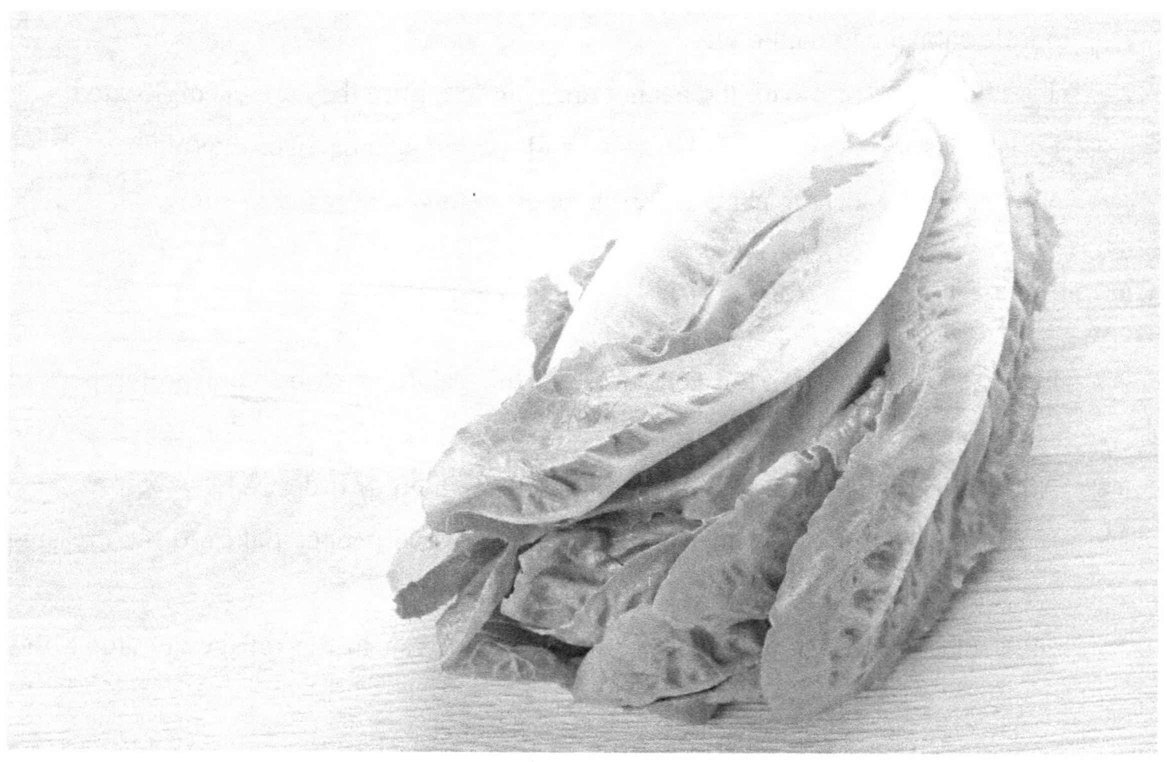

Grilled Romaine Caesar Salad with Herbed White Beans elevates greens. Charred romaine hearts meet creamy Caesar dressing, complemented by tender herbed white beans. This warm and satisfying salad offers a balanced blend of textures and flavors—a creative twist on a classic that's both hearty and refreshing.

Preparation Time: 10 minutes

Cook Time: 35 minutes

Total Time: 45 minutes

Serves:4

Difficulty: Medium

Ingredients:

- 4 large romaine lettuce heads, halved
- 1 cup of cooked white beans
- 2 tablespoons of olive oil
- 1 tablespoon of lemon juice
- 2 cloves of garlic, minced
- 1 teaspoon of Dijon mustard
- 1/4 cup of vegan mayonnaise
- 1/4 cup of nutritional yeast
- 1/4 cup of chopped fresh parsley
- Salt and pepper to taste
- Croutons for serving

Kitchen Tools Needed:

- grill pan
- mixing bowl
- whisk
- knife
- cutting board
- serving platter

xxxxxxxxxxxxxxxxxxx

Instructions:

a. Start by preheating a grill pan over medium-high heat.

b. In a mixing bowl, whisk together the following ingredients to create the dressing: olive oil, lemon juice, Dijon mustard, minced garlic, vegan mayonnaise, nutritional yeast, chopped parsley, salt, and pepper.

c. Brush the halved romaine lettuce heads with the prepared dressing.

d. Place the romaine lettuce halves onto the preheated grill pan and grill for approximately 2-3 minutes on each side, or until they develop a light char.

e. Carefully remove the grilled romaine lettuce from the grill pan and transfer it to a serving platter.

f. In the same mixing bowl used for the dressing, combine the cooked white beans with the remaining dressing.

g. Arrange the herbed white beans evenly over the grilled romaine lettuce.

h. Garnish your salad creation with croutons and an additional sprinkle of chopped parsley.

i. Your Grilled Romaine Caesar Salad with Herbed White Beans is ready to be served immediately.

Cooking Notes:

- To add a protein boost, consider grilling some chicken or tofu to serve alongside this salad.
- Feel free to experiment with different types of beans, such as chickpeas or cannellini beans, for added variety.
- If you prefer a more traditional Caesar salad, you can include grated vegan Parmesan cheese in the dressing.
- This salad pairs beautifully with a crusty baguette or garlic bread on the side.
- To make the croutons, you can cube and toast slices of your favorite bread with a drizzle of olive oil and a sprinkle of garlic powder and herbs.
- Don't overcook the romaine lettuce; a light char adds a delightful smoky flavor while keeping the interior slightly crisp and fresh.

25. Abundance Kale Salad with Savory Tahini Dressing

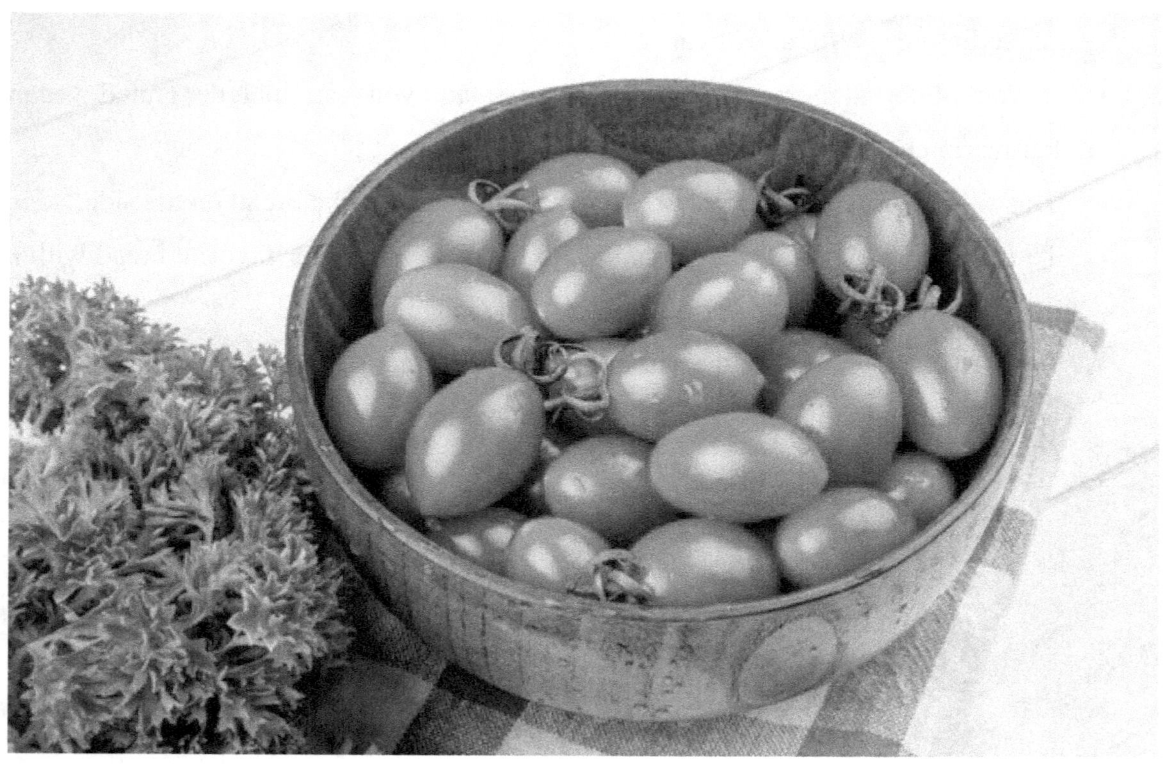

Abundance Kale Salad with Savory Tahini Dressing is a flavor-packed delight. Nutrient-rich kale mingles with an array of vibrant veggies, nuts, and seeds. Drizzled with a savory tahini dressing, this wholesome creation offers a harmonious blend of textures and tastes—a celebration of health and abundance in each bite.

Preparation Time: 10 minutes

Cook Time: 35 minutes

Total Time: 45 minutes

Serves:4

Difficulty: Medium

Ingredients:

- 1 bunch of kale
- 1 cup of cherry tomatoes
- 1 cup of cucumber
- 1 cup of bell peppers
- 1/2 cup of red onion
- 1/4 cup of fresh cilantro
- 1/2 cup of roasted almonds

For the dressing:

- 1/4 cup of tahini
- 2 tablespoons of lemon juice
- 2 tablespoons of olive oil
- 2 cloves of garlic, minced
- 1/2 teaspoon of salt
- 1/4 teaspoon of black pepper
- Water (as needed)

Kitchen Tools Needed:

- Mixing Bowl
- Whisk

Instructions:

a. Begin by thoroughly washing and drying the kale. Afterward, remove the stems and chop the leaves into bite-sized pieces.

b. In a large mixing bowl, combine the chopped kale with cherry tomatoes, cucumber, bell peppers, red onion, cilantro, and roasted almonds.

c. In a separate small bowl, whisk together the tahini, lemon juice, olive oil, minced garlic, salt, and black pepper to create the savory tahini dressing. If the dressing appears too thick, you can gradually add water until it reaches your desired consistency.

d. Drizzle the dressing evenly over the salad and toss everything together until all ingredients are well coated.

e. Allow the Abundance Kale Salad with Savory Tahini Dressing to rest for a few minutes. This helps the flavors meld together for a more delicious result.

f. Serve your vibrant and nutritious kale salad and savor the flavors!

Cooking Notes:

- Massaging the kale leaves with a bit of olive oil and salt before assembling the salad can help soften their texture and reduce bitterness.
- Customize your salad by adding ingredients like avocado, feta cheese, or grilled chicken for extra flavor and protein.
- Store any leftover dressing separately and drizzle it over the salad just before serving to keep it fresh and crisp.
- Feel free to substitute tahini with almond butter or peanut butter for a different flavor twist.
- This salad can be a great side dish or a main course with added protein like grilled tofu or chickpeas.
- Experiment with different nuts or seeds, such as pine nuts or sunflower seeds, for added crunch and nutrition.

26. Rosemary Roasted Root Vegetable Panzanella

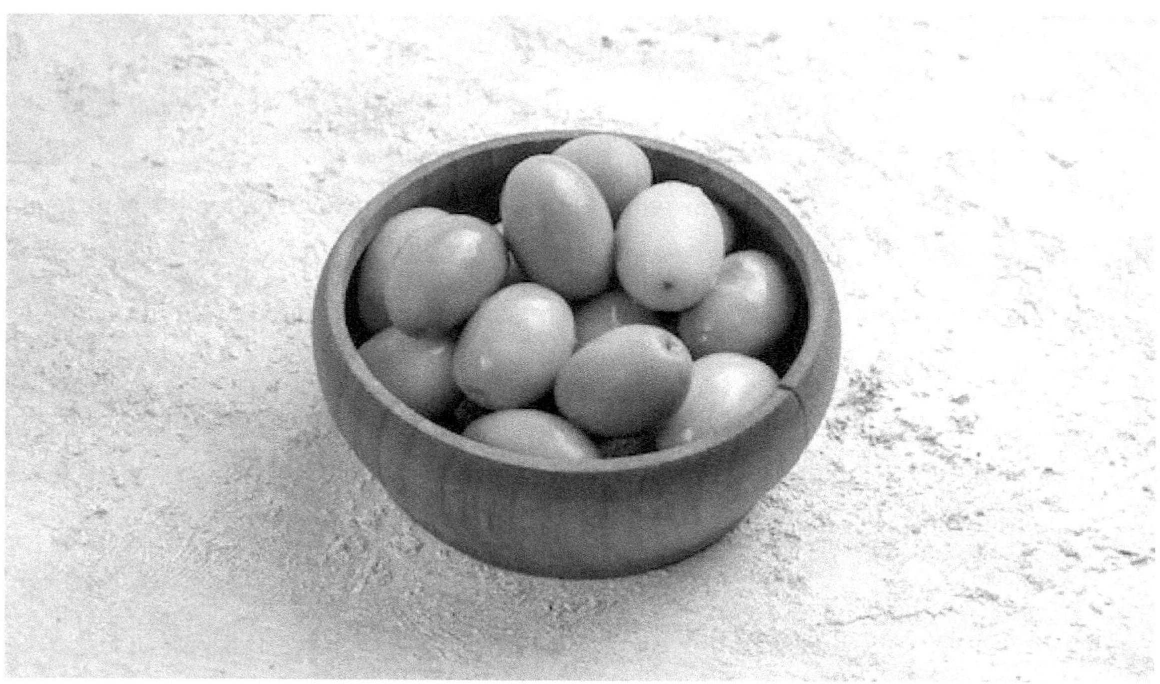

Rosemary Roasted Root Vegetable Panzanella redefines the salad. Colorful roasted veggies meet rustic bread cubes, creating a hearty and flavorful dish. Enhanced with rosemary, it's a warm and aromatic medley that marries textures and tastes, offering a unique and satisfying twist on the traditional panzanella.

Preparation Time: 10 minutes

Cook Time: 35 minutes

Total Time: 45 minutes

Serves:3

Difficulty: Medium

Ingredients:

- 400g of mixed root vegetables (carrots, parsnips, beets, turnips), cut into bite-sized chunks
- 3 tbsp of olive oil
- 1 tsp of dried rosemary
- 1/2 tsp of salt
- 1/4 tsp of black pepper
- 4 cups of stale bread, torn into bite-sized pieces
- 1 cup of cherry tomatoes, halved
- 1/2 cup of red onion, thinly sliced
- 1/4 cup of kalamata olives, pitted and halved
- 2 tbsp of balsamic vinegar
- 1 tbsp of Dijon mustard
- 1 clove of garlic, minced
- 1/4 cup of fresh basil, chopped

Kitchen Tools Needed:

- oven
- baking sheet
- mixing bowl
- whisk

xxxxxxxxxxxxxxxxxxx

Instructions:

a. Start by preheating your oven to 400°F (200°C).

b. In a mixing bowl, combine the root vegetables, 2 tablespoons of olive oil, dried rosemary, salt, and black pepper. Make sure to toss the vegetables thoroughly to ensure an even coating.

c. Spread the prepared vegetables in a single layer on a baking sheet, and then roast them in the preheated oven for about 25-30 minutes. You'll know they're done when they become tender and develop a nice, light browning.

d. In another mixing bowl, assemble the salad components by combining the stale bread, cherry tomatoes, red onion, and kalamata olives.

e. In a separate small bowl, whisk together the remaining 1 tablespoon of olive oil, balsamic vinegar, Dijon mustard, and minced garlic. Pour this flavorful dressing over the bread mixture and give it a good toss to ensure everything is nicely coated.

f. Next, add the roasted root vegetables to the bread mixture and gently toss again, making sure all the ingredients are well combined.

g. Allow the panzanella to rest for about 10 minutes before serving. This will give the flavors a chance to meld together beautifully.

h. Just before serving, garnish your Rosemary Roasted Root Vegetable Panzanella with fresh basil. It can be enjoyed either warm or at room temperature.

Cooking Notes:

- Use a variety of root vegetables like carrots, potatoes, parsnips, and sweet potatoes for a delightful mix of flavors and colors.
- If you don't have stale bread, you can toast fresh bread cubes in the oven for a few minutes until they're slightly crispy.
- Feel free to customize your panzanella with your favorite herbs or additional veggies like bell peppers or cucumbers.
- The bread in panzanella is meant to soak up the delicious dressing, so don't be shy about letting it sit for a bit before serving.
- You can make this dish ahead of time, but it's best to add the bread and fresh basil just before serving to maintain their texture and flavor.
- Serve your Rosemary Roasted Root Vegetable Panzanella as a hearty side dish or add some grilled chicken or tofu to make it a complete meal.

27. Chickpea Chopped Kale Salad with Adobo Dressing

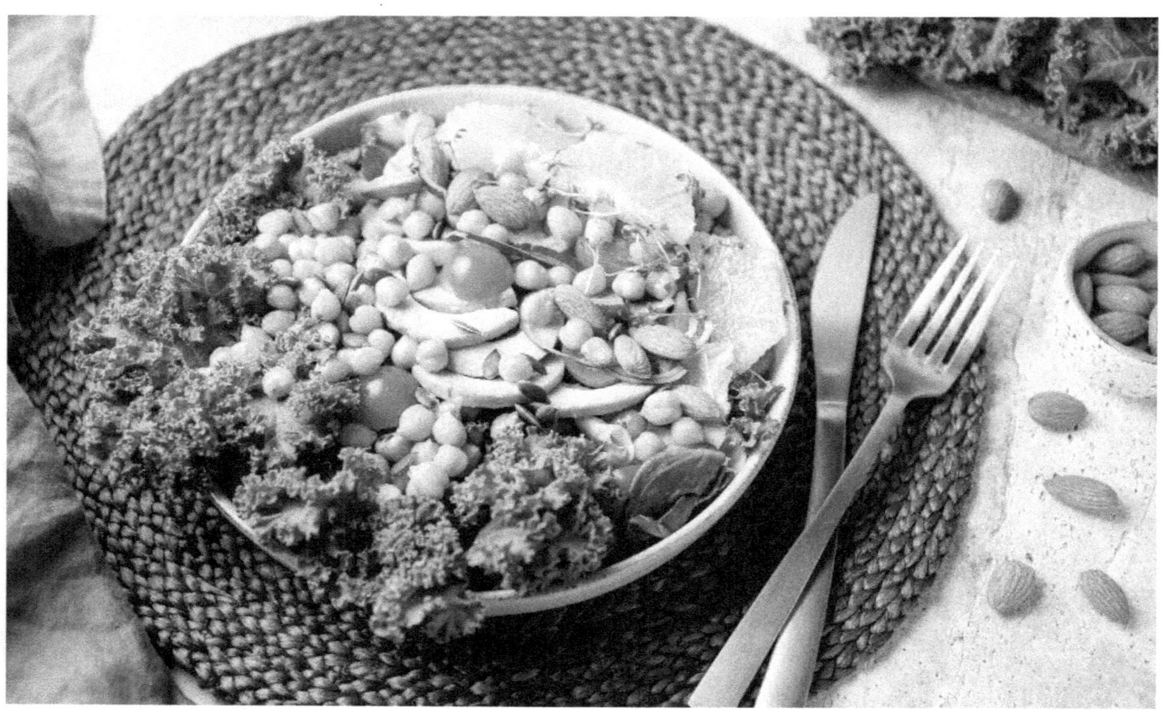

Chickpea Chopped Kale Salad with Adobo Dressing is a bold fusion. Robust adobo-spiced chickpeas meet chopped kale, offering a satisfying crunch. Drizzled with a zesty dressing, this hearty salad celebrates both savory and healthful elements—a flavor-packed and nutrient-rich culinary adventure in every bite.

Preparation Time: 10 minutes

Cook Time: 35 minutes

Total Time: 45 minutes

Serves:3

Difficulty: Medium

Ingredients:

- 3 cups of kale, chopped
- 1 can (15 oz) of chickpeas, drained and rinsed
- 1/2 cup of halved cherry tomatoes
- 1/4 cup of finely sliced red onion
- 1/4 cup of chopped roasted red peppers
- 1/4 cup of pitted and sliced olives
- 2 tbsp of chopped fresh parsley
- 8 tablespoons of chopped fresh basil
- 1 tbsp of fresh lemon juice
- a half teaspoon of garlic powder
- smoked paprika, 1/2 tsp
- 1/2 tablespoon of cumin
- 1 tablespoon of salt
- 1/4 teaspoon of ground black pepper
- 2 tbsp of olive oil
- 1 teaspoon of apple cider vinegar
- 1 tsp of maple syrup
- 1/2 teaspoon of chipotle adobo sauce (from a can)

Kitchen Tools Needed:

- mixing bowl
- whisk

Instructions:

a. In a large bowl, combine the chopped kale, chickpeas, cherry tomatoes, red onion, roasted red peppers, pitted olives, parsley, and basil.

b. In a small bowl, whisk together the lemon juice, garlic powder, smoked paprika, cumin, salt, black pepper, olive oil, apple cider vinegar, maple syrup, and adobo sauce.

c. Pour the dressing over the salad and toss to combine.

d. Allow the salad to sit for at least 15 minutes to let the flavors meld together.

e. Serve the Chickpea Chopped Kale Salad with Adobo Dressing either as a standalone dish or as a flavorful side.

Cooking Notes:

- You can customize this salad by adding ingredients like grilled chicken, feta cheese, or avocado for added protein and richness.

- Adjust the level of adobo sauce to suit your spice preference. Add more for extra heat or less for a milder flavor.

- To make this salad in advance, keep the dressing separate until just before serving to maintain the kale's crispness.

- Massaging the kale leaves with a bit of olive oil and salt before adding the other ingredients can enhance their texture and flavor.

- This salad is an excellent choice for meal prep as it keeps well in the refrigerator for a day or two, making it a convenient and healthy lunch option.

28. Cheesy Roasted Broccoli & Chickpea Kale Salad

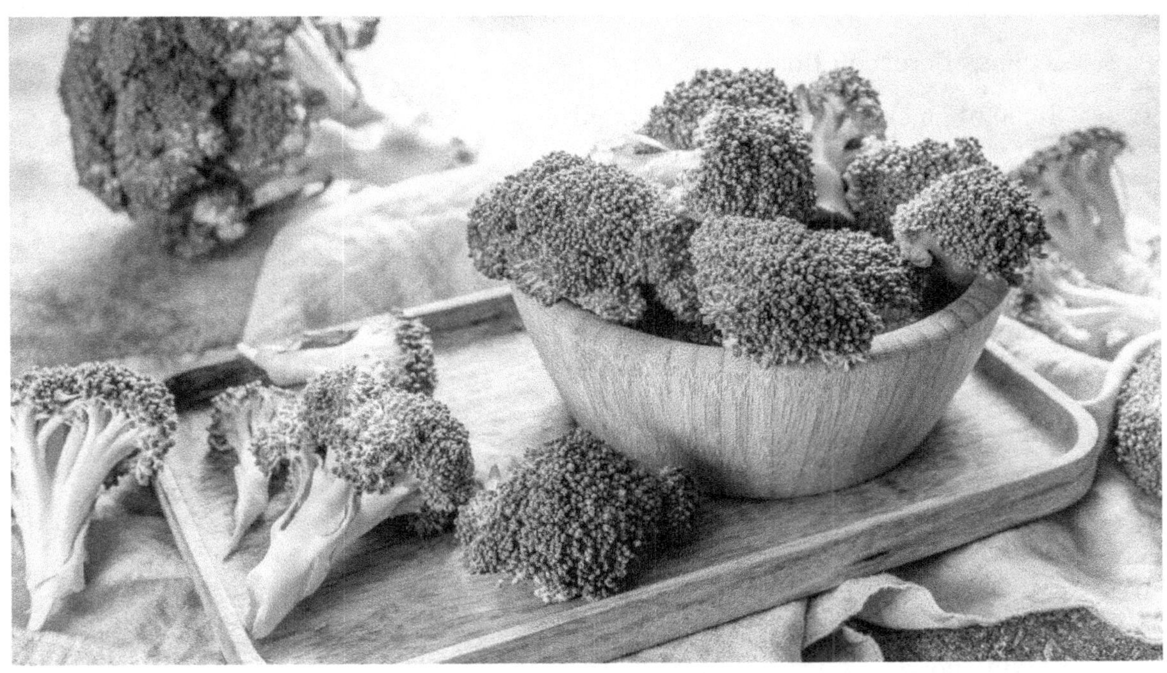

Cheesy Roasted Broccoli & Chickpea Kale Salad is a taste sensation. Nutty chickpeas and charred broccoli join chopped kale, drizzled with a cheesy dressing. This flavorful and nutritious salad offers a medley of textures and tastes, creating a satisfying and wholesome dish that's both indulgent and health conscious.

Preparation Time: 10 minutes

Cook Time: 35 minutes

Total Time: 45 minutes

Serves: 3

Difficulty: Medium

Ingredients:

- 3 cups of broccoli florets
- 1 can of chickpeas, drained and rinsed
- 4 cups of kale, chopped
- 1/4 cup of nutritional yeast
- 1/4 cup of olive oil
- 2 tablespoons of lemon juice
- 2 cloves of garlic, minced
- Salt and pepper to taste

Kitchen Tools Needed:

- Baking sheet
- Mixing bowl
- Whisk

XXXXXXXXXXXXXXXXXXXX

Instructions:

a. In a large bowl, combine the chopped kale, chickpeas, cherry tomatoes, red onion, roasted red peppers, pitted olives, parsley, and basil.

b. In a small bowl, whisk together the lemon juice, garlic powder, smoked paprika, cumin, salt, black pepper, olive oil, apple cider vinegar, maple syrup, and adobo sauce.

c. Pour the dressing over the salad and toss to combine.

d. Allow the salad to sit for at least 15 minutes to let the flavors meld together.

e. Serve the Chickpea Chopped Kale Salad with Adobo Dressing either as a standalone dish or as a flavorful side.

Cooking Notes:

- You can customize this salad by adding ingredients like grilled chicken, feta cheese, or avocado for added protein and richness.

- Adjust the level of adobo sauce to suit your spice preference. Add more for extra heat or less for a milder flavor.

- To make this salad in advance, keep the dressing separate until just before serving to maintain the kale's crispness.

- Massaging the kale leaves with a bit of olive oil and salt before adding the other ingredients can enhance their texture and flavor.

- This salad is an excellent choice for meal prep as it keeps well in the refrigerator for a day or two, making it a convenient and healthy lunch option.

- Feel free to experiment with different herbs and greens, such as cilantro or spinach, to suit your taste.

29. Masala Chickpea Stuffed Sweet Potatoes

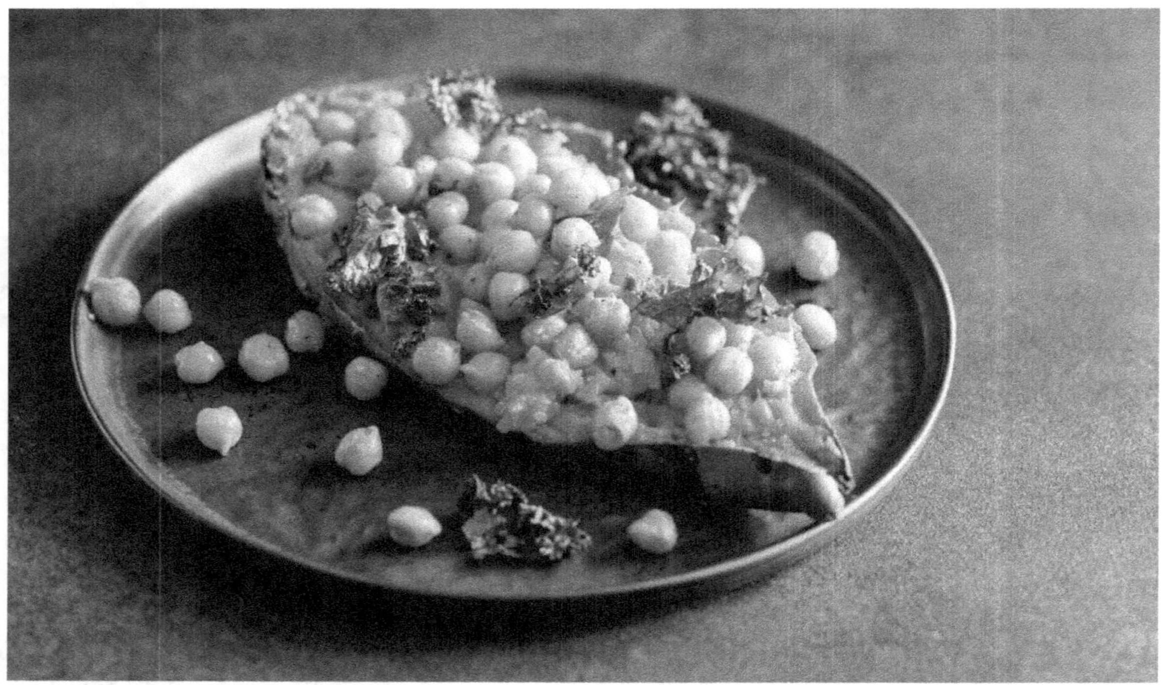

Masala Chickpea Stuffed Sweet Potatoes redefine comfort. Roasted sweet potatoes are filled with spiced chickpeas, creating a flavorful and satisfying dish. Bursting with Indian-inspired flavors, this plant-based creation offers a harmonious blend of textures and tastes—a fusion of healthfulness and indulgence in each bite.

Preparation Time: 10 minutes

Cook Time: 35 minutes

Total Time: 45 minutes

Serves: 4

Difficulty: Medium

Ingredients:

- 4 medium sweet potatoes
- 1 can (400g) of washed and drained chickpeas
- 1 tablespoons of olive oil
- 1 small, sliced onion
- 2 minced garlic cloves
- 1 teaspoon of cumin powder
- 1 teaspoon of coriander powder
- 8 teaspoon of turmeric powder
- 1/2 teaspoon of paprika powder
- A half teaspoon of salt
- 1/4 teaspoon of ground black pepper
- 1/2 cup of spinach, chopped
- 1/4 cup of fresh cilantro, chopped
- 1/2 lemon juice

Kitchen Tools Needed:

- oven
- baking sheet
- mixing bowl
- whisk

XXXXXXXXXXXXXXXXXXX

Instructions:

a. Preheat the oven to 400°F (200°C).

b. In a mixing bowl, combine the broccoli florets, chickpeas, nutritional yeast, olive oil, minced garlic, salt, and pepper. Ensure everything is well coated.

c. Spread the mixture on a baking sheet and roast for 25-30 minutes, until the broccoli is tender and lightly browned.

d. While the broccoli and chickpeas are roasting, prepare the kale by massaging it with lemon juice and a pinch of salt for a few minutes until it begins to soften.

e. Once the roasted broccoli and chickpeas are done, set them aside to cool slightly.

f. In a large bowl, combine the roasted broccoli, chickpeas, and massaged kale. Toss everything together to combine.

g. Serve the salad as a main course or as a side dish. Enjoy!

Cooking Notes:

- You can customize this salad by adding your favorite toppings like cherry tomatoes, sliced avocado, or a sprinkle of seeds or nuts.

- For extra flavor, consider drizzling a light dressing made from olive oil, lemon juice, and your preferred seasonings.

- Massaging the kale helps to tenderize it and reduce its bitterness, making it more enjoyable in salads.

- Don't overcook the broccoli; it should be tender but still slightly crisp.

- This salad can be served warm or at room temperature, depending on your preference.

- Feel free to experiment with different seasonings or cheese varieties to suit your taste.

30. Butternut Squash & Miso Brussels Sprouts Nourish Bowl

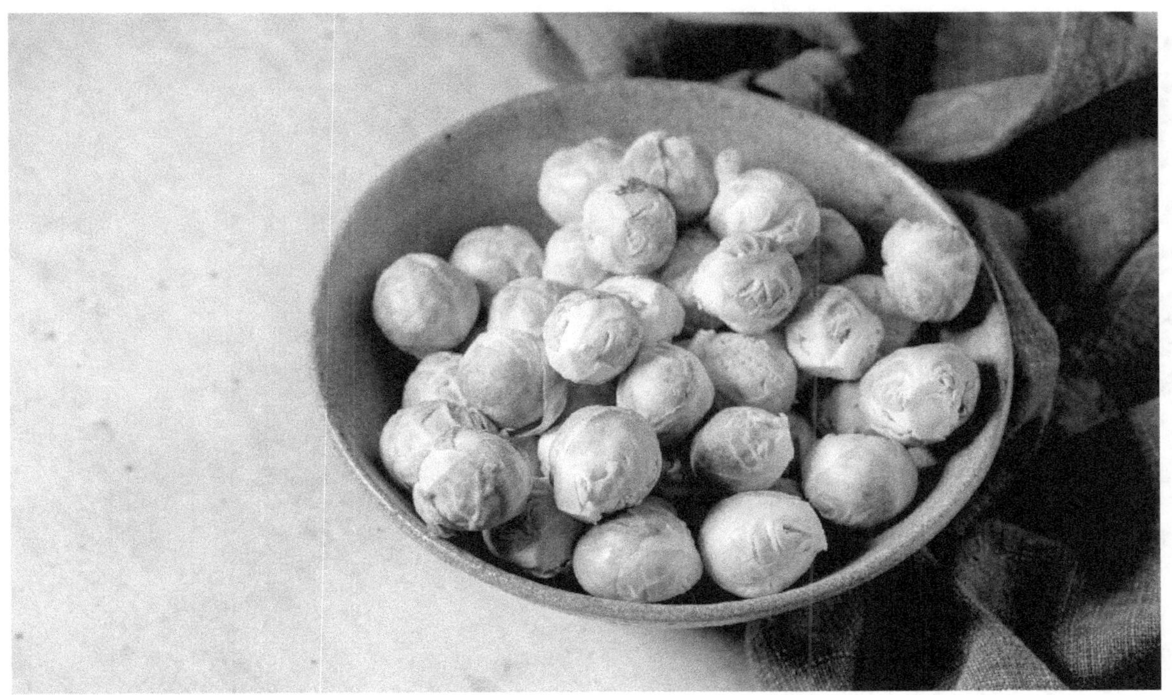

Butternut Squash & Miso Brussels Sprouts Nourish Bowl is a wholesome delight. Roasted butternut squash meets miso-glazed Brussels sprouts, creating a flavorful and nourishing base. Topped with grains, greens, and seeds, this vibrant bowl offers a balanced blend of textures and tastes—a comforting and healthful culinary experience.

Preparation Time: 10 minutes

Cook Time: 35 minutes

Total Time: 45 minutes

Serves: 3

Difficulty: Medium

Ingredients:

- 1 butternut squash, peeled and cubed
- 1 pound of Brussels sprouts, trimmed and halved
- 2 tablespoons of miso paste
- 2 tablespoons of maple syrup
- 2 tablespoons of soy sauce
- 2 tablespoons of rice vinegar
- 1 tablespoon of sesame oil
- 2 cups of cooked quinoa
- 1 cup of edamame beans, cooked
- 1 avocado, sliced
- 1/4 cup of sesame seeds

Kitchen Tools Needed:

- oven
- baking sheet
- mixing bowl
- whisk

xxxxxxxxxxxxxxxxxxxx

Instructions:

a. Preheat the oven to 425°F (220°C).

b. In a large bowl, combine the butternut squash, Brussels sprouts, miso paste, maple syrup, soy sauce, rice vinegar, and sesame oil. Mix well to evenly coat the vegetables.

c. Arrange the vegetable mixture in a single layer on a sheet of parchment paper.

d. Roast in the preheated oven for 25-30 minutes, or until the vegetables are tender and slightly caramelized.

e. In the meantime, cook the quinoa following the package instructions.

f. Once the vegetables and quinoa are cooked, divide the quinoa evenly among three bowls.

g. Top each bowl with the roasted vegetables, edamame beans, avocado slices, and sesame seeds.

h. Serve the nourishing bowls warm and enjoy!

Cooking Notes:

- Customize your nourish bowl with additional toppings like roasted nuts, crumbled feta cheese, or a drizzle of tahini for added flavor and texture.
- You can prepare a large batch of roasted vegetables and store them in the refrigerator for quick and easy bowl assembly during the week.
- Feel free to substitute quinoa with other grains like brown rice, farro, or couscous according to your preference.
- Make the miso dressing ahead of time and store it separately for convenient use on various salads and bowls.
- Experiment with different vegetables based on what's in season for a fresh and diverse flavor profile.
- These nourish bowls are versatile and can be adapted to suit various dietary preferences, such as vegan, vegetarian, or gluten-free, by choosing appropriate ingredients and dressings.

Conclusion

As our flavorful journey through Fiber-Rich Feasts comes to a close, we invite you to continue embracing the wonderful synergy of taste and health that high-fiber foods offer. From the hearty crunch of vegetables to the comforting embrace of whole grains, these recipes have shown us that nourishing our bodies can be a vibrant and joyful experience. Remember, Fiber-Rich Feasts are more than just recipes; they represent a lifestyle that prioritizes wellness without compromising on flavor or creativity. By weaving high-fiber ingredients into your meals, you're not only supporting your digestive health but also fostering a deeper connection with the food you enjoy.

Whether you're exploring new culinary horizons or simply seeking to enrich your menu with nutrient-rich goodness, Fiber-Rich Feasts empower you to create a symphony of taste and wellness on your plate. Here's to savoring each bite, embracing a health-conscious approach, and embarking on a path where nourishment and enjoyment walk hand in hand.

Thank you – Thank you – Thank you

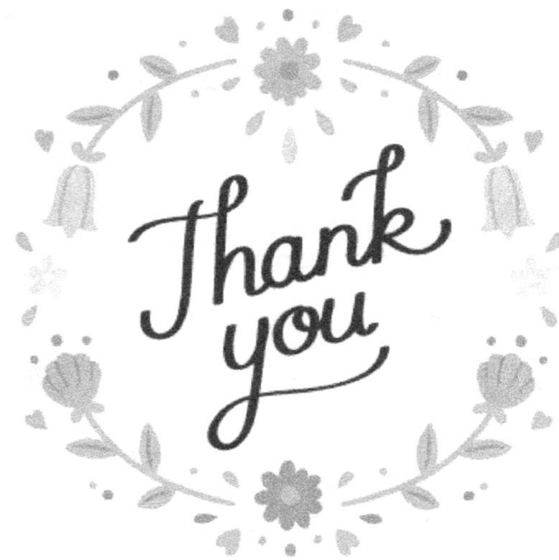

I am grateful to you for purchasing and reading my book. It brings me great joy to write, and my motivation stems from my desire to help others. Writing allows me to achieve this goal, and I am grateful for the opportunity to do so.

May I ask what led you to choose this particular book? With so many books and authors exploring similar topics, it means a lot that you chose mine. Your decision is truly appreciated, and I am confident that you will find the book to be immensely beneficial.

I would love to hear your thoughts on the book. As authors, we grow and improve based on the feedback we receive from our readers. Even a small comment or review would be greatly appreciated. Your feedback could even serve as inspiration for other readers. Thank you once again for your support.